Laboratory Investigation of Endocrine Disorders

Laboratory Investigation of

Endocrine Disorders

Second Edition

Michael R. Wills RD, MD, PhD, MRCP, FACP, FRCPath
Director of Clinical Laboratories, University of Virginia Medical Center,
Charlottesville, Virginia, USA
Formerly Professor and Director of the Metabolic Unit, Royal Free Hospital, London

Bill Havard MA, DM, FRCP
Physician in Charge of the Endocrine Unit, Royal Free Hospital, London

Butterworths
London Boston Durban Singapore Sydney Toronto Wellington

First published, 1979
Second edition 1983

© Butterworth & Co (Publishers) Ltd 1983

British Library Cataloguing in Publication data

Wills, Michael R.
    Laboratory investigations of endocrine disorders.
    —2nd ed.
    1. Endocrine gland—Diseases—Diagnosis
    2. Diagnosis, Laboratory
    I. Title   II. Havard, Bill
    616.4′075   RC649

    ISBN 0–407–00276–6

Library of Congress Cataloging in Publication Data

Wills, M. R. (Michael Ralph)
    Laboratory investigations of endocrine disorders.

    1. Endocrine glands—Diseases—Diagnosis.
2. Hormones—Analysis. 3. Diagnosis, Laboratory.
I. Havard, C. W. H. (Cyril William Holmes)
II. Title. III. Title: Endocrine disorders.
[DNLM: 1. Diagnosis, Laboratory. 2. Endocrine
diseases—Diagnosis.   WK 100 W741L]
RC649.W54   1983   616.4′0756   83-2651
ISBN 0–407–00276–6

Typeset by Scribe Design, Gillingham, Kent
Printed and bound by Whitefriars Press Ltd, Tonbridge, Kent

Preface to the Second Edition

The need for a Second Edition of this book within three years of publication of the First Edition confirms the need for a basic guide to the available endocrine laboratory tests. In this edition the original text has been revised and two additions have been made. A new chapter has been added which deals with disorders of calcium homeostasis and their investigation with particular reference to hypercalcaemia and hypocalcaemia. An Appendix has been included which contains a set of normal endocrine reference values and also the factors for the conversion of numerical values in 'old' or conventional units to those in the 'new' SI system. It is, however, important to recognize that reference values are affected by many variables. Among the latter the most important are the assay technique and the age and sex of the patient. The reference values given in the Appendix should, therefore, only be used as general guidelines and a diagnostic or therapeutic decision should be based on the reference values provided by the laboratory that has done the assay.

Michael R. Wills
Bill Havard

Preface to the First Edition

In the past decade there has been a vast increase in the number of laboratory tests that are available for the investigation of patients with endocrine disorders. This has occurred simultaneously with considerable developments in the understanding of the mechanisms involved in the pathogenesis of these disorders. Regrettably, all too often in the investigative process there has been some misuse of the laboratory tests as patients with endocrine disorders represent only a small proportion of the whole medical spectrum. The objective of this manual has been to provide senior clinical students and medical practitioners, in all grades and specialties, with a basic guide to the endocrine laboratory tests that are available; not only when to do which test but also precisely how to do it as well as recognizing its limitations. The manual should also be of value to the laboratory-based scientist, both the medical and the non-medical, as a standardized basis on which to provide advice to the laboratory user. In each section the basic physiology on which the investigations are based has been provided in order to give a rational basis for their usage. Although the normal range and reference values may vary slightly between individual laboratories, because of methodological variations, the tests and the protocols that we have described are all well established and non-controversial.

Michael R. Wills
Bill Havard
Peter J. Roylance

Contents

6. Disorders of the adrenal medulla   61

7. Ovarian disorders   65

Appendix

1 Thyroid disorders

Physiology

The thyroid gland secretes its principal hormones, thyroxine (T_4) and tri-iodothyionine (T_3) into the circulation where they are associated with two proteins (the thyroxine-binding proteins) that bind them specifically. By paper electrophoresis the proteins appear between the α_1 and α_2 globulins (thyroxine-binding globulin (TBG)) and ahead of the albumin (thyroxine-binding pre-albumin (TBPA)); in addition, a minor fraction of the hormone is bound to albumin itself. In the bound form, thyroxine and tri-iodothyronine are distributed throughout the extracellular fluid and are measurable by chemical or immunochemical assay.

T_3 is the metabolically active form of thyroid hormone. Nevertheless T_3 measurements cannot be substituted for T_4 measurements in the clinical assessment of thyroid function for a number of reasons. Eighty per cent of the circulating T_3 is derived from de-iodination of T_4 by peripheral tissues so that T_3 is only an indirect reflection of thyroid secretion. Stress, starvation and systemic illness decrease the rate of de-iodination so that the serum T_3 level may be normal in the sick hyperthyroid patient. Furthermore the suppression of thyroid-stimulating hormone (TSH) is more dependent on circulating levels of T_4 than of T_3 so that in iodine deficiency, for example, the TSH may be raised because the circulating concentration of T_4 is low but the patient is euthyroid because the levels of T_3 are normal. Similarly, adequate T_3 replacement therapy of the hypothyroid patient may not suppress TSH secretion in contrast to adequate T_4 replacement therapy.

Both T_4 and T_3 are largely bound to plasma proteins. In the case of T_4 99.95% is bound and with T_3 99.5%. It is the free hormone that is metabolically active. Changes in the concentration of the serum binding protein will lead to parallel changes in the serum values of total thyroid hormones, but the free thyroid hormone values remain constant.

The control of thyroid hormone secretion is complex. A tripeptide thyrotrophin-releasing hormone (TRH) is synthesized and stored in the median eminence of the hypothalamus. It is released into the portal veins of the pituitary stalk. In the anterior pituitary it promotes pulsatile release of the glycoprotein TSH. It also promotes the release of prolactin although the physiological significance of this is at present unknown.

Thyrotrophin, the circulating concentration of which shows some nyctohemeral variation, stimulates most metabolic processes in the thyroid from iodide uptake to release of thyroid hormones. The mechanism is probably that thyrotrophin binds to a receptor site on the thyroid cell membrane and activates adenyl cyclase. This leads to a cyclic adenosine monophosphate (AMP) mediated activation of one or more enzymes ultimately leading to an increased release of T_4 and T_3 into serum.

In iodide deficiency states, and in conditions where thyroid throughput is accelerated, there is a relative switch in thyroid synthesis from the less active T_4 to the more active T_3. This could represent a control mechanism or could be explained on purely synthetic grounds since T_3 contains one less iodine atom and is one step less complex than T_4.

Specimens and normal range values

For all the thyroid hormone assays and antibodies 10 ml of venous blood should be sent to the laboratory in a sterile container.

Most of the *in vitro* tests attempt to measure the concentrations of the circulating thyroid hormones in the blood (T_4 and T_3). These hormones circulate in the plasma bound to proteins, particularly TBG. In the interpretation of laboratory results it is important to recognize those factors or diseases which may affect the concentration of TBG, and thus the assayed hormone concentration, although the actual amount of free hormone may not have changed.

Factors altering TBG are as follows:

Factors Reducing TBG

Nephrosis
Acromegaly
Corticosteroids
Malnutrition
Androgens and anabolic steroids
Old age

Factors Increasing TBG

Pregnancy
Oestrogens
Clofibrate (Atromid-S)
Phenothiazines

Factors Reducing Binding Capacity of TBG

Renal failure,
Drugs bound to TBG such as:
    Salicylates
    Phenytoin (Epanutin)
    Phenylbutazone
    Fenclofenac

Total serum thyroxine (T$_4$)

The normal range of T$_4$ for adults is 54–142 nmol/ℓ. Values up to 240 nmol/ℓ are found in neonates, in pregnancy and in patients on the contraceptive pill; other than these variations there is little change with either age or sex.

The assay is useful in the diagnosis of both hyperthyroidism and hypothyroidism.

There are, however, a number of causes for a discrepancy

between the measured serum T_4 and the patient's true thyroid status, as outlined below:

1. Change in serum concentration of TBG.
2. Drugs binding to TBG.
3. Disease states altering binding properties of TBG.
4. Conditions altering the ratio of T_3 to T_4, such as:
    Iodine deficiency
    Patients treated with T_4
    Patients treated with ^{131}I
    Patients with chronic thyroiditis
    T_3 thyrotoxicosis

Total serum tri-iodothyronine (T₃)

The normal range of T_3 for adults is 0.8–2.5 nmol/ℓ with higher values being obtained in the neonatal period and in pregnancy. Males tend to have slightly lower levels than females. As with T_4, values for T_3 are affected, although to a lesser extent, by variations in the concentration of binding proteins.

The assay of T_3 is of value in the special situation of a patient who is suspected of having T_3-thyrotoxicosis when the T_4 value may be normal. This situation is rare and represents less than 5% of all thyrotoxic patients in the United Kingdom.

Free binding capacity (FBC) (normal range 90–105%)

The abbreviation FBC should be used instead of the earlier term 'T_3 resin uptake'. This assay provides an indirect measurement of the unoccupied thyroxine-binding protein sites available in the patient's serum. It does not give any information about total serum T_3 value and is unaffected by iodine contamination. It should *only* be used in conjunction with a measurement of serum T_4 to calculate the free thyroxine index.

Free thyroxine index (FTI) (normal range 53–142)

The FTI is obtained from the measurement of serum T_4 and FBC. It is an attempt to obtain an indirect measurement of free thyroxine. The scientific validity of this index is debatable as the index is relative (results are related to a normal control) and is imprecise (containing two ratios). The FTI is of value in returning T_4 results from euthyroid pregnant (or on the contraceptive pill) patients back to the normal adult range. Misleading results can occur, particularly in the thyroid assessment of elderly patients. The free thyroxine index is also less reliable in acute non-thyroidal illness, when it is often subnormal in the presence of a normal or even high free thyroxine level.

Thyrotrophin (TSH)

The reference range for normal adults varies slightly between centres but is usually from a lower detection limit of 1 mU/ℓ–6 mU/ℓ. Levels may be higher in neonates. A significant elevation (usually to at least 10 mU/ℓ) is found in primary hypothyroidism. Most existing assays are subject to cross-reaction problems to a small extent either from other glycoprotein hormones with similar structure or from other proteins. A few patients who are otherwise clinically and biochemically euthyroid have moderate or high apparent thyrotrophin levels. This may be caused by cross-reaction or may reflect early or latent hypothyroidism ('subclinical hypothyroidism').

In vivo tests

In vivo tests involve the administration of radioiodide (or ^{99m}Tc as pertechnetate which behaves similarly) to patients. Uptake measurements are obtained from serial neck counting, which give an idea of the trapping and hormonal incorporation of iodide. Scanning the thyroid after radioiodide administration shows the distribution of function in the thyroid gland.

20 minute thyroid uptake using intravenous ^{99m}Tc (normal range 0.4–3.0%)

This test is a measure of the ability of the thyroid to concentrate iodide as reflected in ^{99m}Tc uptake. Normal results occur in 5–10%

of thyrotoxic patients. Conversely, patients with non-toxic goitre may have raised values.

Thyroid scan

Indications for scanning are as follows:

1. Identification of aberrant thyroid tissue; lingual thyroid, intrathoracic goitre.
2. Nodular goitre; identification of hot and cold nodules.
3. Thyroid cancer:
   (*a*) To ascertain whether surgical removal has been complete after thyroidectomy
   (*b*) To determine whether recurrent nodules or lymph nodes concentrate radioiodine
   (*c*) To discover whether distant metastases concentrate radioiodine

Thyrotrophin-releasing hormone (TRH) test

TRH was the first hypothalamic releasing hormone to be made commercially available in a synthetic form. This compound provides a dynamic *in vivo* method for the assessment of thyroid function and also pituitary function. TRH does not usually stimulate the release of either growth hormone (GH), adrenocorticotrophic hormone (ACTH) or the posterior lobe hormones, but it does have a consistent effect on prolactin (*see* page 18) and has a variable effect on luteinizing hormone (LH) and follicle-stimulating hormone (FSH) release.

Side-effects   Following the rapid intravenous injection of TRH there may be mild and transient side-effects: nausea, slight dizziness, peculiar taste, facial flushing, sensation of heat and desire to micturate. These have been attributed to a contractile effect of TRH on smooth muscle. The test should *only* be used in patients with chronic obstructive airway disease or asthma, and in patients with ischaemic heart disease if considered to be an essential procedure.

Patient preparation   The TRH response is diminished in patients receiving corticosteroids or thyroid hormones, and is enhanced after oestrogen treatment (in males) and following over-treatment with antithyroid drugs and with theophylline. Treatment with thyroxine should be stopped for at least three weeks, and with tri-iodothyronine and corticosteroids for at least two weeks prior to the test.

Method
1. Zero time–collect venous blood sample.
2. Give 200 µg of synthetic TRH in 2 ml of physiological saline solution as a rapid intravenous injection.
3. 20 minutes after injection–collect venous blood sample for TSH.
4. 60 minutes after injection–collect venous blood sample for TSH.

Normal response   Typically, the TSH concentration increases to a peak response of between 5 and 20 mU/ℓ at 20 minutes and then falls to one-third of the peak response at 60 minutes.

Females tend to have a greater response when compared with males, probably due to their higher circulating oestrogen concentration. Their response is also greater in the pre-ovulatory phase of the menstrual cycle when compared with post-ovulation.

In both males and females there is greater response at night than during the day and TRH tests should be done at a standardized time of day.

Age, height, weight and surface area are reported not to affect the TRH response.

Causes of a flat TRH response in biochemically euthyroid patients   Among such causes are the following:

Treated thyrotoxicosis	Patients taking thyroxine in
Ophthalmic Graves' disease	excess of 0.15 mg daily
Non-toxic nodular goitre	Cushing's syndrome
Simple goitre	Hypopituitarism
Autonomous nodule	Acromegaly
	Idiopathic

In advanced renal or hepatic disease the response to TRH may be delayed and the elevation in TSH prolonged.

Exaggerated and prolonged TRH response   Primary hypothyroidism.

> *Note*: This test is useful diagnostically in hypothyroidism, readily distinguishing between primary thyroid hypofunction and hypothyroidism secondary to pituitary disease. It is important to recognize, however, that in most clinical situations the assay of serum TSH is adequate for the diagnosis of primary hypothyroidism. The TRH test is also a sensitive indicator of hyperthyroidism when the results of routine tests are inconclusive; an absent response is found in patients with T_3 thyrotoxicosis.

Other tests

Thyroid antibodies in thyroiditis

When thyroid auto-antibodies develop, they are of two main types: those directed against thyroglobulin, and those against a microsomal fraction of thyroid cells. Thyroglobulin antibodies from patients with chronic thyroiditis react with all normal colloid extracts and with all thyrotoxic glands but not with abnormal forms of thyroglobulin made in dyshormonogenetic goitres, and to a minor extent in all longstanding nodular colloid goitres. The microsomal antigen is a lipoprotein in the membrane of the small vesicles which contain newly synthesized thyroglobulin on its way to the colloid. Thyrotoxic glands contain about 10 times the normal amount of the microsomal antigen in keeping with their increased synthetic activity. Thyroid cancers contain little or no microsomal antigen, and show a poor radioactive iodine uptake and impaired hormone synthesis.

Thyroid antibody tests are of value in the diagnosis of chronic thyroiditis and in the management of Graves' disease. Both antithyroglobulin and microsomal antibodies must be measured since they may be found together or separately in any one serum.

In patients suspected of hypothyroidism, the presence of thyroid antibodies supports the diagnosis and may even ante-date the development of any significant clinical evidence of thyroid failure.

Note: It is important to remember that some normal subjects and patients with other auto-immune conditions (particularly pernicious anaemia) may also have these antibodies.

Thyroid-stimulating antibodies (TSAb)

The hyperthyroidism of Graves' disease is due to antibody production to the TSH-receptors in the thyroid cell membrane. Some of the antibodies fit the receptor precisely and mimic all the effects of TSH. Other antibodies fit the receptor less precisely and provoke only some of the effects of TSH. These antibodies are called thyroid-stimulating antibodies to distinguish them from the more familiar destructive antibodies of Hashimoto's disease and chronic thyroiditis. Some antibodies like the long-acting thyroid stimulator (LATS) have no effect on the human gland but stimulate the thyroid in certain animal species. Other antibodies like LATS protector stimulate the human gland but not that of the animal. The name LATS protector' was given because IgG from thyrotoxic sera, inactive in the LATS assay, can block the absorption of LATS by thyroid microsomes *in vitro* because it contains another antibody, LATS protector. This blocking antibody is human-specific and is almost certainly responsible for the thyroid stimulation in Graves' disease.

TSAbs are auto-antibodies made in lymphoid cells and combined with TSH receptors where they activate the adenyl cyclase/cyclic adenosine monophosphate system at the cell surface.

Note: Assays for LATS and LATS protector are not routinely available.

Cholesterol

Cholesterol is a non-specific measurement of end-organ response to thyroid hormones, high serum levels being characteristic of hypothyroidism. *It is diagnostically useless.*

Diagnostic considerations

Hypothyroidism

Hypothyroidism is the clinical condition resulting from decreased circulating concentrations of free (unbound) thyroid hormones. Clinical features include sensitivity to cold, lack of energy, dry skin and a hoarse voice. Hypothyroidism is commonly due to primary thyroid failure when serum thyrotrophin concentration is high due to a lack of negative feedback at the pituitary level by thyroid hormones. It can also be secondary to pituitary failure of thyrotrophin secretion when serum thyrotrophin values are usually low or just within the normal range.

If there are clinical signs of hypothyroidism the assay of total serum thyroxine is the most useful single biochemical test. Results below 50 nmol/ℓ confirm hypothyroidism and below 20 nmol/ℓ are usually indicative of primary hypothyroidism. Results in the range 50–70 nmol/ℓ may be considered borderline and thyrotrophin estimation is necessary. Primary hypothyroidism is usually associated with a basal thyrotrophin of at least 10 mU/ℓ.

It is important to remember that it is possible for an individual to be euthyroid when the serum T_4 is low because of adequate T_3 production. There are several situations when there is a sequential failure of first T_4 production and later T_3. Examples of this include patients who have received ^{131}I therapy and individuals with chronic thyroiditis.

If thyroxine and thyrotrophin results are borderline, or if there is a possibility of pituitary thyrotrophin deficiency, a TRH test is useful. An exaggerated response of thyrotrophin to TRH confirms primary hypothyroidism; a subnormal or delayed response is compatible with pituitary or hypothalamic dysfunction. As thyrotrophin deficiency is often associated with deficiency of other pituitary hormones the latter must then be investigated.

Thyroid antibodies are a useful secondary test in hypothyroidism. Chronic thyroiditis, a common cause of primary hypothyroidism, is associated with antibodies present in high titre. Total serum tri-iodothyronine is often within the normal range in primary hypothyroidism but is low in a variety of acute and chronic non-thyroid illnesses. It is therefore *of no value in the diagnosis of hypothyroidism.*

Perchlorate discharge test

The test is used to identify organification defects in the synthesis of thyroxine. Perchlorate blocks the trapping of iodine by the gland and if dyshormogenesis is present unbound iodine will diffuse out of the gland. If the synthesis of thyroxine is normal, no such loss of iodine will occur.

Side-effects   No side effects from a single dose of perchlorate have been reported.

Patient preparation   The patient should be fasted from food and fluids overnight for a minimum of 12 hours. The patient should not have received anti-thyroid drugs, thyroxine or iodine-containing drugs for the previous four weeks.

Method
1. Zero time–a tracer dose of radioactive iodine (^{123}I, ^{131}I, ^{132}I) is given by mouth.
2. 60 minutes after dose of tracer, the iodine uptake over the thyroid is measured.
3. Immediately after uptake measurement – potassium per-chlorate 600 mg is given by mouth.
4. 90 minutes after the dose of iodine – the iodine uptake over the thyroid is measured.
5. 120 minutes after the dose of iodine – the iodine uptake over the thyroid is measured.

Normal response   There should normally be a fall of thyroid radioactive iodine uptake of less than 10% at 90 or 120 minutes after the dose of iodine. A greater fall is indicative of a defect in the organification of iodine.

Hyperthyroidism

Hyperthyroidism is the clinical condition resulting from increased circulating serum concentrations of free thyroid hormones.

Symptoms include weight loss, heat intolerance, tachycardia and lid retraction. The main causes of hyperthyroidism are Graves' disease, toxic multinodular goitre, toxic nodule, painless thyroiditis and trophoblastic TSH syndrome, but the condition can be induced by over-treatment with thyroid hormones.

Total serum tri-iodothyronine is a sensitive indicator of hyperthyroidism and in most cases is raised to a much greater extent than total serum thyroxine. It may be the only thyroid hormone elevated. The incidence of 'T$_3$-toxicosis' (hyperthyroidism with elevated T$_3$ but normal T$_4$) varies between centres, but is on average less than 5% of hyperthyroid patients in the United Kingdom. The condition may be related to dietary iodide deficiency and may also reflect early hyperthyroidism. Total serum T$_4$ is less discriminating than T$_3$ since it is not so sensitive; however, serum T$_4$ is successful in detecting the majority of hyperthyroid patients.

When T$_4$ and T$_3$ results are borderline there is a choice of diagnostic strategies. For pregnant patients in whom *in vivo* tests may be contra-indicated, and others who are thought to have abnormal binding proteins, the FTI index may be of value. Alternatively, a dynamic function test gives more useful information. An impaired or absent TSH response in a TRH test is suggestive of hyperthyroidism.

In vivo uptake tests can, however, be performed rapidly and are elevated in the majority of patients with hyperthyroidism. Increasing contamination of the environment with iodine has reduced the

Table 1.1. Summary of tests in hypothyroidism and hyperthyroidism

	First choice test	Confirmatory tests	Tests to provide more information
In primary hypothyroidism*	T$_4$	TSH	Thyroid antibodies
In secondary hypothyroidism*	T$_4$	TRH test	Other pituitary function tests
In hyperthyroidism†	T$_4$	T$_3$ ^{99m}Tc uptake TRH test	

*In hypothyroidism uptake tests are not helpful.
†In patients who are either pregnant or on the contraceptive pill, the only measurement of value is the FTI or, if hypothyroidism is suspected, the TSH.

importance of *in vivo* tests. If the inorganic iodine stores of the body are increased there is a decrease in the uptake of the isotope. Iodine is a constituent of health foods such as kelp; iodine compounds are used as colouring materials for drugs and foods. The use of iodine contrast media in radiology is steadily increasing. A thyroid scan after radioisotope administration is useful to distinguish the diffuse goitre characteristic of Graves' disease from nodular goitres. The main application of the thyroid scan is in the detection of cold nodules.

Investigation of thyroid status in patients after treatment of hyperthyroidism

Three methods of treating hyperthyroidism are widely used; antithyroid drugs; radioactive iodine; and partial thyroidectomy. These treatments have a risk of either recurrent hyperthyroidism or of developing hypothyroidism months or years later. Life-long follow-up should always be undertaken.

At follow-up visits the patient should be examined clinically for features of hyperthyroidism or hypothyroidism. Which biochemical tests are of value in long-term follow-up is open to some debate. The total serum T_4 appears to be the most useful single test. Total serum T_3 is of some value for suspected recurrent hyperthyroidism but the results must be interpreted with caution since T_3 values can remain high during treatment, particularly with antithyroid drugs such as carbimazole. Thyrotrophin is a very sensitive indicator of developing hypothyroidism, revealing incipient thyroid failure weeks or months before T_4 results drop below the normal range.

Investigation of thyroid status in patients after treatment of hypothyroidism

The treatment of choice for hypothyroidism is thyroxine as a single daily dose of 100–200 µg. When patients are started on this replacement therapy it is advisable to measure serum TSH concentrations soon after starting on a low dose to check that values have fallen to within the normal range. Subsequently, the clinical assessment of the patient and measurement of serum T_4 may be used to check adequacy of treatment; T_4 results greater than 100 nmol/ℓ confirm the latter. An elevated serum T_3 provides biochemical confirmation of over-replacement. If patients are receiving treatment with T_3 then measurement of the serum T_4 will give a misleading impression of their thyroid function. Patients who are euthyroid on T_3 medication will have low levels of T_4 as their TSH production will be suppressed and their endogenous production of T_4 will be minimal. If there is clinical evidence of inadequate treatment, or if it is not certain if medication is being taken regularly, then the serum TSH is the most sensitive biochemical indicator. However, when a patient is taken off an adequate dose of thyroxine after long-term treatment, some months may elapse before pituitary thyrotrophin secretion reestablishes itself and T_4 estimations are most useful.

2 Hypothalamic–anterior pituitary disorders

Physiology

The hypothalamus is involved in the control of the activities of the functionally distinct anterior and posterior lobes of the pituitary gland.

The hormones secreted by the pituitary glands are as follows:

Anterior pituitary	Posterior pituitary
Growth hormone (somatotrophin) –GH	Vasopressin
Adrenocorticotrophin hormone –ACTH	Oxytocin
Prolactin–PRL	Neurophysin
Thyrotrophin or thyroid-stimulating hormone–TSH	
Follicle-stimulating hormone–FSH	
Luteinizing hormone–LH	
These hormones are synthesized and released from the cells of the anterior pituitary under the influence of the hypothalamic-releasing or inhibiting hormones.	These hormones are synthesized in hypothalamic nuclei and only stored in the posterior lobe.

The hypothalamic hormones synthesized in hypothalamic neurones are stored in nerve endings in the median eminence from which they are released into the hypophyseal venous portal plexus and are thus transported to their target cells in the anterior lobe of the pituitary. The secretion rates of the hypothalamic

Table 2.1 Principal stimuli affecting hormone secretion rates

Hormone	Normal secretion increased by	decreased by
Growth hormone (GH)	Stress and fear Exercise Early phase of sleep Amino acids (arginine) Bovril Blood sugar fall Glucagon Dopamine	Hyperglycaemia Fatty acids Excess corticosteroids
Prolactin	Stress Lactation Late and early phases of sleep	
Luteinizing hormone (LH)	Males: fall in testosterone* Females: sudden rise in oestrogen*	Males: rise in testosterone* Females: sustained rise in oestrogen*
Follicle-stimulating hormone (FSH)	Males: low sperm count* Females: low oestrogen*	Females: high oestrogen*
Thyroid-stimulating hormone (TSH)	Fall in tri-iodo-thyronine or thyroxine	Rise in tri-iodo-thyronine or thyroxine
Adrenocorticotrophin (ACTH)	Stress Blood sugar fall* Fall in cortisol*	Quiet conditions Rise in cortisol*

*Stimuli acting predominantly or entirely at pituitary level.

hormones are influenced by environmental stimuli and negative feedback control from the products of the target organs of the anterior pituitary hormones, some of which (for example, thyroxine) also act at the pituitary level. In the interpretation of assayed hormone concentrations, in the diagnostic situation, it is essential to be aware of the principal stimuli affecting the hormone secretion rates, as listed in *Table 2.1*.

Specimens and normal range values

For the assay of GH, PRL, LH, FSH and TSH – 5 ml samples of venous blood should be sent to the laboratory in sterile containers.

Growth hormone

Basal plasma values of GH are normally low throughout the day, being less than 10 mU/ℓ and may often be undetectable; the values may be higher in children than in adults. In normal subjects, however, transient peaks in plasma GH do occur which are of a spontaneous nature, and unrelated to the presence of those factors which normally affect the secretion rate. It is essential to use provocative tests to demonstrate a deficiency of GH, but the finding of one high value proves that a deficiency does not exist.

Follicle-stimulating and luteinizing hormones

In females FSH stimulates development and maturation of the ovarian follicles and ova, although there is also some requirement for LH. The developing follicle secretes oestrogen in increasing amounts. At mid-cycle the rise in oestradiol operates a positive feedback effect, unique to females, and a short burst of extra LH is induced which releases the ovum from the ripened follicle and promotes the conversion of the latter into the progesterone-secreting corpus luteum. A longer lasting or greater rise in oestradiol activates the more usual negative feedback effect on LH secretion.

Table 2.2 Normal range values for FSH and LH

	FSH (U/ℓ)	LH (U/ℓ)
Females		
Follicular phase	3–16	3–45
Mid-cycle phase	12–27	45–300
Luteal phase	2–16	3–45
Post-menopausal	40–185	49–128
Males	3–16	5–23
Children – 1 year to puberty	2.5	—

In males FSH causes spermatogenesis within the seminiferous tubules, and LH (sometimes called the interstitial cell-stimulating hormone (ICSH)) stimulates the interstitial cells to secrete testosterone.

Normal range values are as shown in *Table 2.2*.

Prolactin

PRL is similar in size and structure to GH and like the latter it is also secreted in response to stress, in short spontaneous bursts during a normal day under basal conditions, and particularly during the early and late phases of sleep. There is also a physiological variation through the day in normal subjects with lower values in the afternoon when compared with the forenoon. Prolactin is unique in being the only pituitary hormone primarily controlled by an inhibiting hormone (PIH) rather than by a releasing hormone. PIH is almost certainly dopamine. Prolactin values are higher during the ovulatory and luteal phases of the menstrual cycle than during the follicular phase. There is a progressive increase in prolactin values during pregnancy to reach a maximum at the end with values of the order of 17 times the mean value in non-pregnant females. In lactation the mechanical stimulation of suckling itself leads to an increase in prolactin values in the immediate post-partum period. Prolactin values do, however, decrease, despite persistent lactation, and reach basal values between 3 to 7 weeks after delivery.

Normal range values are:

Females   25–396 mU/ℓ
Males   5–178 mU/ℓ

Various factors are able to increase prolactin concentration; these include oestrogens, thyrotrophin-releasing hormone (TRH) and various stress situations such as hypoglycaemia following insulin injection. Likewise, substances which inhibit PIH secretion lead to an increased release of prolactin into the circulation. They include a number of psychotropic drugs, which either block the effects of dopamine or cause dopamine depletion in nervous structures, in particular in the hypothalamus, and also the contraceptive pill. Drugs that block the effects of dopamine include the phenothiazines, butyrophenone and metoclopramide. Drugs that deplete brain stores of dopamine include reserpine and methyldopa.

The measurement of prolactin concentration is useful in determining the involvement of this hormone in the causation of amenorrhoea and galactorrhoea, and is thus the basis for logical treatment with an inhibitor of its secretion, such as bromocryptine. Prolactin concentration is not increased in all cases of functional galactorrhoea. This is probably due to the fact that the production and ejection of milk is a complex process in which several reflex, metabolic and endocrine factors are involved amongst which prolactin secretion is merely one component. In galactorrhoea associated with a pituitary adenoma, prolactin values are very frequently raised. In patients with normal values these could be explained by the episodic secretion of a prolactin producing adenoma; in such a situation serial values through a 24-hour cycle may be of value.

The measurement of prolactin is also of value in the investigation of amenorrhoea as approximately 25% of patients with secondary amenorrhoea have increased prolactin concentrations. It is one of the most important investigations in infertility.

Adrenocorticotrophin

Assay of ACTH is *not* routinely available. If the assay is to be undertaken then it is *essential* that a strict protocol is rigidly followed; a number of factors can influence the plasma concentration (particularly stress in any form); ACTH is adsorbed onto glass, it is also very unstable in whole blood and is destroyed by proteolytic enzymes present in serum and plasma.

Although no specific patient preparation is required, basal samples should be collected at around 0900 hours with, in addition, a further sample at around 2400 hours if it is intended to assess the nyctohemeral rhythm. In many situations only a single sample is necessary.

Approximately 15 ml of venous blood should be collected into a plastic syringe, without stress, and then immediately transferred into a pre-cooled heparin containter (plastic), taken to the laboratory surrounded by ice and separated, preferably at 4°C within ten minutes of collection.

The only clinical situations where an ACTH assay may be of value are as follows:

1. To establish the causative mechanism in a patient with proven Cushing's syndrome, as distinct from diagnosing the condition. Where the syndrome is due to an adrenal adenoma or

carcinoma, ACTH will not be detectable, whereas markedly raised values will be found in patients with non-endocrine hormone-secreting tumours, and high normal or slightly raised values in patients with adrenal hyperplasia due to pituitary causes (basophil adenoma).
2. To differentiate between primary and secondary adrenocortical failure.
3. To assess the adequacy of treatment in patients with Cushing's syndrome or with the adrenogenital syndrome.

Dynamic tests

Insulin stress test *see* page 34

Tetracosactrin test *see* page 32

LH–RH test

In the normal adult, the intravenous administration of 25–100 µg of gonadotrophin-releasing hormone LH/FSH–RH (LH–RH) causes a rapid dose-dependent increase in serum LH and a smaller increase in FSH.

In females, after doses of 100 µg, there is a rise in oestradiol levels. Near the mid-cycle LH peak and during the luteal phase, the LH response to releasing hormone is greater than in the follicular phase–possibly due to an increased circulating concentration of oestradiol and progesterone. It seems that steroids sensitize the pituitary to respond to LH–RH with a selective augmented release of gonadotrophins.

In the male, the gonadotrophin responses are the same as in the female, but are insufficient to cause statistically significant changes in the serum levels of the gonadal steroid hormones, testosterone or oestradiol, or in their precursors (17-hydroxy-progesterone or progesterone). The LH–RH, therefore, causes both LH and FSH release in man but does not affect growth hormone, thyrotrophin or ACTH in the normal individual.

The LH–RH test provides a measure of the functional integrity of the hypothalamic–pituitary–gonadal axis, although it may not provide definite information with respect to the actual site or extent of a lesion.

Diagnostic value

Females In the female, the LH–RH test has been used to evaluate several disorders affecting the hypothalamic and/or pituitary gland presenting with menstrual disturbances or infertility. If gonadotrophin values are unequivocally elevated there is no need to proceed to an LH–RH test. If, however, they are normal to low, some information on pituitary function may be obtained with an LH–RH test. It has, however, been suggested that there is no certain way to differentiate primary hypothalamic from pituitary failure, and that in such a situation a single assay of LH and FSH may provide as much information as the LH–RH test. Although the test alone may not distinguish between pituitary and hypothalamic causes of hypogonadism it is possible by combining it with a clomiphene stimulation test to effect a functional separation which may be useful in treatment.

Some of these conditions may be associated with hyperprolactinaemia and/or galactorrhoea. In this instance, the problem becomes one of hyperprolactinaemia.

Hypothalamic–pituitary disorders in which the LH–RH test may be of value in females are as follows:

1. Organic hypothalamic lesions.
2. Isolated hypogonadotrophic hypogonadism.
3. Post-operative assessment following hypophysectomy.
4. Polycystic ovaries (Stein–Leventhal syndrome).
5. Primary amenorrhoea.
6. Secondary amenorrhoea:
   (*a*) Without galactorrhoea
         anorexia nervosa
         malnutrition
         iatrogenic (including 'post-pill')
         idiopathic
         psychogenic
         post-traumatic
         post-partum
         pituitary tumours, including lesions of the stalk
   (*b*) With galactorrhoea
         iatrogenic (including 'post-pill')

idiopathic
non-post-partum
post-partum
pituitary tumours, including lesions of the stalk

Males   In the male the LH–RH test is of value in the investigation of Hypogonadotrophic hypogonadism as follows:

1. Primary:
adult
pubertal
cryptorchism

2. Secondary (with or without oligospermia or azoospermia):
iatrogenic
psychogenic
systemic diseases
traumatic
idiopathic
tumours (acromegaly, Cushing's syndrome)
infection (tuberculosis, meningitis, etc.)
pituitary ablation

Method

Table 2.3 Schedule for LH–RH test

Time (min)	Action
−3	(Basal) Collect venous blood for LH and FSH
0	Inject 0.1 mg of LH–RH intravenously
+20 +60	Collect venous blood for LH and FSH

Normal response

Table 2.4 Normal response for LH–RH test

	Time	LH (U/ℓ)	FSH (U/ℓ)
Female (follicular phase)	Basal	3–45	3–16
Male	Basal	5–23	3–16

Note: Basal values are variable depending on the stage of the menstrual cycle. After LH–RH the LH values should increase eight-fold and the FSH values double.

Disease state responses

1. An exaggerated response with initial high basal values indicates primary gonadal failure.
2. A poor response may indicate a hypothalamic or pituitary disorder.
3. A normal response does not exclude a hypothalamic disturbance.

Combined test

In suspected pituitary or hypothalamic lesions it is possible to do the TRH, LH/FSH–RH and insulin stress tests simultaneously. Venous blood samples are collected for basal values of glucose, cortisol, GH, TSH, LH and FSH. At zero time insulin, TRH and FSH/LH–RH, Relefact, (one ampoule contains 100 µg LH–RH and 200 µg TRH) are injected immediately one after the other. Subsequent venous blood samples are then collected at the appropriate times for the individual tests. This combined test offers an almost complete evaluation of anterior pituitary function.

Diagnostic considerations

Hypopituitarism

It is usual for there to be a deficiency of most, if not all, of the anterior pituitary hormones. In pituitary or hypothalamic disorders there is usually a progressive sequence of loss of the hormones of the anterior lobe, with associated clinical disturbances. The usual progression is shown in *Table 2.5*.

Unless there has been either surgical damage or trauma to the pituitary stalk it is rare to have associated deficiency of neurohypophyseal hormones.

There may be single hormone deficiency states due to the simple lack of the appropriate releasing factor; these are usually congenital.

Table 2.5 Progressive sequence of loss of pituitary hormones

Hormone	Clinical effects	
LH, FSH	In females:	Oligomenorrhoea
		Amenorrhoea
		Infertility
	In males:	Impotence
		Azoospermia
		Decrease in size and softening of testes
	In both sexes:	Decreased libido
		Loss of sexual hair
		Fineness and wrinkling of skin
GH	Impairment of growth in children	
PRL	Failure of lactation	
TSH	Hypothyroidism	
ACTH	Adrenocortical insufficiency without pigmentation	

The principal lesions associated with hypopituitarism are as follows:

1. Pituitary tumours (adenomas): chromophobe, eosinophil, basophil.
2. Hypothalamic or stalk tumours: metastatic lesions (particularly from breast and lung), local tumours such as craniopharyngioma, meningioma, pinealoma, glioma and hamartoma.
3. Infections, granulomas and infiltrations: tuberculous basal meningitis, sarcoidosis, syphilis, encephalitis, histiocytosis-X, haemachromatosis, non-tuberculous giant cell granuloma.
4. Vascular lesions: post-partum necrosis (Sheehan's syndrome), severe hypotension following haemorrhage, vascular malformations in hypothalamus.
5. Iatrogenic conditions: surgical ablation, radiation, yttrium implantation, selective failure of TSH or ACTH after prolonged therapy with equivalent hormone.
6. Trauma: head injury with or without fracture of the base of the skull.

The insidious progressive nature of the loss of anterior lobe hormones means that patients may present with the full clinical picture of hypopituitarism or with partial deficiency states. The diagnosis of the latter must be made with the following specific dynamic *in vitro* tests:

1. LH, FSH deficiency–poor response in the LH/FSH–RH test.
2. GH deficiency – insulin stress test (*see* page 34).
3. ACTH deficiency – a low 0900-hour plasma cortisol concentration associated with some response to tetracosactrin (*see* page 33). The cortisol response will depend on the severity of the secondary adrenal atrophy.
4. PRL deficiency–prolactin levels can be followed either during an insulin stress test or a TRH test (*see* pages 34 and 6). The value of dynamic tests is, however, debatable.

Growth hormone excess

An excess of GH causes gigantism if it occurs before epiphyseal fusion, and acromegaly if it occurs after that event. The excess of secretion is usually due to an eosinophil, a chromophobe or a mixed cell pituitary adenoma. To some degree the adenoma remains under hypothalamic control; it is possible that the basic defect in acromegaly and gigantism is prolonged and inappropriate hypothalamic stimulation of the pituitary, caused either by excess secretion of GH-releasing hormone or deficiency of GH release-inhibiting hormone. The pituitary tumour may be associated with increased activity of other endocrine glands in the pluriglandular syndrome. These syndromes may be familial and show an autosomal dominant inheritance.

Acromegaly
The clinical features include soft-tissue overgrowth with exaggerated skin folds, carpal tunnel syndrome, skeletal overgrowth (especially of the skull, hands and feet), osteoarthrosis, excessive sweating, goitre, diabetes mellitus, hypertension, headache and gynaecomastia. Visual field defects such as bitemporal hemianopia occur if the tumour extends out of the pituitary fossa.

The diagnostic biochemical features are:

1. Resting plasma GH more than 10 mU/ℓ.
2. Failure of GH to suppress to less than 2 mU/ℓ after an oral 50 g glucose load with successive blood sampling for glucose and

GH at 30-minute intervals for 2½ hours. The actual values may vary from 20 mU/ℓ to over 100 mU/ℓ and there is often a paradoxical rise instead of a fall in serum GH following the glucose load. In patients with severe hepatic or renal disease a rise in blood glucose may also not depress serum GH concentration.

Associated biochemical features which are found in some patients include:

1. Impaired glucose response in an oral glucose tolerance test (a 'diabetic' glucose tolerance curve).
2. Hypercalciuria.
3. Hypercalcaemia.
4. Hypopituitarism.

Gigantism

Excessive secretion of GH before the epiphyseal plates of the long bones and vertebrae have fused results in gigantism. These giants have normal body proportions, with an arm span equal to their height. The metabolic complications are the same as in acromegaly and the patient will eventually develop acromegalic features. In the diagnosis of gigantism the main problem is the differentiation of patients with growth hormone excess from those who are constitutionally tall. The latter often have a family history, show normal serum GH concentrations and suppression of GH to values of less than 2 mU/ℓ following an oral glucose load.

Galactorrhoea

Excessive prolactin secretion usually results in inappropriate lactation, especially in breasts sensitized by exposure to normal or increased amounts of oestrogens or progestogens. It is much more common in females than males and is usually accompanied by amenorrhoea, oligomenorrhoea or impotence and infertility. The patients are often overweight. It may accompany the amenorrhoea that sometimes follows oral contraceptive therapy. Occasionally, galactorrhoea and amenorrhoea with hyperprolactinaemia may occur in association with hypothyroidism.

A common cause of galactorrhoea is the administration of drugs, and may be divided as follows:

1. Drugs that block the effects of dopamine:
        Phenothiazines
        Butyrophenone (Haloperidol)
        Metoclopramide (Maxolon)
2. Drugs that deplete brain stores of dopamine:
        Reserpine
        Methyldopa
3. Oestrogens (contraceptive pill)

Other causes are:

1. Hypothalamic–pituitary disease:
        Chromophobe adenoma, macrodenoma or microadenoma
        Acromegaly
        Post-hypophysectomy
        Cushing's disease
2. Hypothyroidism.

Clinically, the galactorrhoea is accompanied by excess fat in the breast but not much glandular hyperplasia, which occurs more characterically in oestrogen-dependent gynaecomastia such as occurs at puberty, after oestrogens, or in men with oestrogen-secreting testicular or adrenocortical tumours. The accompanying hypogonadism is not the result of deficient gonadotrophins since serum FSH and LH concentrations are usually normal, but may be due to inhibition of the actions of the gonadotrophins on the gonad by the raised prolactin concentration. Many patients with hyper-prolactinaemia have gonadal dysfunction – amenorrhoea, oligomenorrhoea or impotence – without clinically obvious lactation.

The indications for serum prolactin assay are:

1. Galactorrhoea.
2. Amenorrhoea.
3. Infertility.
4. Menstrual abnormalities.
5. Hypothalamic—pituitary disease.

Precocious puberty

Excessive secretion of gonadotrophins in a child may lead to precocious puberty. The cause may be constitutional or the result of a brain lesion. The condition must be distinguished from pseudo-precocious puberty, in which a patient develops premature secondary sexual characteristics without maturation of the gonads; pseudo-puberty results from excessively high concentrations of gonadal steroids coming from either the adrenals or the ovaries or testes (for example, tumours or congenital adrenal hyperplasia) and the patients are infertile.

Clinically, the patients show acceleration of skeletal growth with the development of secondary sexual characteristics. Constitutional precocious puberty is much more common in girls than boys; the usual cause of precocious puberty in boys is a hypothalamic tumour.

Biochemically, adult levels of gonadotrophins will be present in the blood of patients with precocious puberty but are suppressed in pseudo-puberty.

3 Hypothalamic–pituitary–adrenocortical axis

Physiology

Adrenal cortical function is largely under the control of the (anterior) pituitary *adrenocorticotrophic hormone (ACTH)*. Secretion of ACTH is normally subjected to three variables: nyctohemeral rhythm*, a feedback mechanism; and response to stress. The nyctohemeral rhythm is dependent on the individual's sleeping habits. It results in cyclical changes in ACTH secretion with consequent variations in corticosteroid production (*cortisol* and *corticosterone*), usually producing the highest circulating blood concentrations at about the time of waking with the lowest values during the early sleep period. The feedback mechanism is a negative one in that a rise in plasma cortisol concentration acts on the hypothalamus to inhibit the pituitary release of ACTH. In response to physical, psychological or metabolic stress (for example, pain, fear, hypoglycaemia) there is an increase in ACTH and corticosteroid secretion which can obliterate the influences of both the nyctohemeral rhythm and the feedback mechanisms. All three variables act predominantly through the hypothalamus which produces a neuro-hormone, *corticotrophin releasing factor (CRF)*, which is carried to the cells of the anterior pituitary gland in hypothalamic–hypophyseal portal vessels. CRF stimulates ACTH release from the anterior pituitary. It is on an understanding of this overall physiological control system that the interpreta-

*The preferred term to either circadian or diurnal rhythm

tion of tests of hypothalamic–pituitary–adrenal function depends.

Cortisol is the most important steroid secreted by the adrenal cortex and estimation of its plasma concentration provides the basis for most tests of adrenocortical function. Cortisol circulates in plasma in a protein-bound form. Normally, about 80% is bound to a specific binding α-globulin (*transcortin*) and some of the remainder is loosely bound to albumin. When plasma cortisol values are in the physiological range only a small proportion (approximately 10%) remains free. The transcortin binding sites become saturated when the plasma cortisol concentration exceeds approximately 280 nmol/ℓ and the amount of free cortisol then increases rapidly. Free cortisol is regarded as the biologically active fraction. Methods for plasma cortisol estimation measure the total; that is, both the free and the bound cortisol. With increased or decreased transcortin concentrations the total plasma cortisol may be increased or decreased although the biologically active free cortisol fraction is normal. Transcortin production by the liver is increased by oestrogens and decreased in liver disease; it is lost in the urine in patients with the nephrotic syndrome. Progesterone displaces cortisol from its binding sites on transcortin.

ACTH is a straight chain polypeptide containing 39 amino acids. Its biological activity resides in the first 24 amino acids (N-terminal end) and this part of the molecule is common to most species. Immunological activity resides in the rest of the molecule.

Specimens and normal range values

Plasma cortisol

A 10 ml venous blood sample should be collected into a heparin or plain tube. Sepcimens should be taken to the laboratory immediately after collection for separation. If a delay in separation is unavoidable (for example, a midnight sample) the specimen should be stored at 4°C.

Urine for steroids

24-hour collections for 17-oxogenic and oxosteroids should be in special containers to which have been added 1 ml of 10% methiolate or 4 g of boric acid.

Urine for free cortisol estimation should be collected in a plain bottle and sent to the endocrine laboratory immediately after completion of the collection period.

Urine 17-oxogenic steroids – measures glucocorticoids
Urine 17-oxosteroids – measures androgens
Urine-free cortisol – measures 11 hydroxycortico-steroids (cortisol)

Note: The patient should be off all drugs if at all possible while these tests are done as a wide range of compounds cause interference.

Table 3.1 Normal range values

	0900h	2400h
Plasma cortisol	220–770	55–250 nmol/ℓ
Urine 17-oxosteroids*		
Adult female		14 – 60 µmol/24h
Adult male		20 – 90 µmol/24h
Urine 17-oxogenic steroids*		
Adult female		14 – 50 µmol/24h
Adult male		17 – 70 µmol/24h
Urine free cortisol		
Adult female		216 – 860 nmol/24h
Adult male		300 – 1100 nmol/24h
or		
8h overnight excretion = 25–220 nmol		

*There is a variation in the urine excretion of both steroids with age. Urine 17-oxosteroids and oxogenic steroids are not a reliable index in differentiating Cushing's syndrome from simple obesity.

Dynamic tests

The estimation of plasma cortisol is of most value when used in conjunction with procedures that directly or indirectly stimulate or suppress the adrenal cortex. In this context, the test procedures may be divided into three groups as follows:

1. The adrenal response to exogenous ACTH: tetracosactrin tests.

2. Ability to produce ACTH in response to various stimuli:
   (*a*) hypoglycaemia (insulin stress test)
   (*b*) fall in plasma cortisol (metyrapone test)
   (*c*) lysine vasopressin
   (*d*) artificial fever (pyrogen test)
   Of these, the insulin stress test is the safest, the least unpleasant and most informative. The pyrogen and the lysine vasopressin tests are now obsolete. The metyrapone test is rarely used. All these tests assume a normal adrenal response to endogenous ACTH.
3. Ability to reduce ACTH output in response to a raised plasma cortisol level: dexamethasone suppression tests.

The sites of action of these various test procedures are shown in *Figure 3.1*.

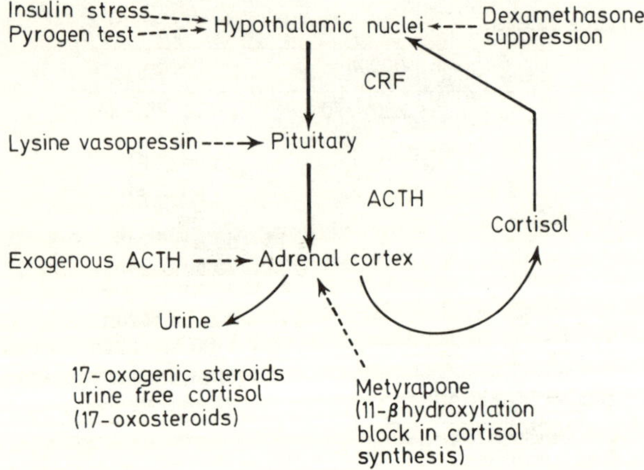

Figure 3.1 Investigation plan showing the sites of action of various test procedures

Tetracosactrin

Natural endogenous ACTH is a straight chain polypeptide containing 34 amino acids. Tetracosactrin is a compound identical with the first 24 amino acids of ACTH. It possesses the adrenocortical stimulatory actions of ACTH, and causes an immediate and maximal adrenal response. Its use has superseded the old exogenous ACTH stimulation test in the investigation of patients with suspected adrenocortical insufficiency.

Short tetracosactrin test

Method   A control blood sample must be taken for plasma cortisol, preferably at about 0900 hours, followed by 250 μg of tetracosactrin intramuscularly. Further blood samples for plasma cortisol should be taken 30 minutes and 60 minutes after giving the tetracosactrin (actual times should be recorded on the laboratory request form and on the specimens).

> *Note:* Certain drugs interfere with plasma cortisol measurement.

Interpretation   The basal level of plasma cortisol should be greater than 200 nmol/ℓ, with an increment of at least 200 nmol/ℓ after the administration of tetracosactrin. The final level should be greater than 500 nmol/ℓ irrespective of the basal level. All three criteria should be fulfilled in a normal response.

Long test

Method   Urinary 17-oxogenic steroid or free cortisol levels are determined on complete 24-hour collections for five consecutive days. The first two days serve as a control period. The subject is then given once daily intramuscular injections of 1 mg of tetracosactrin depot for the remaining three days.

Interpretation   In normal subjects urinary 17-oxogenic steroid or free cortisol excretion at least doubles on the first day of tetracosactrin depot stimulation and continues to increase during the remainder of the test. The long tetracosactrin test offers advantages over the short test only in differentiating between primary and secondary adrenocortical insufficiency. No response is found in patients with the primary type (Addison's disease) whereas with prolonged stimulation in the great majority of patients there is a marked but delayed corticosteroid response in secondary adrenal atrophy. Thus, a marked increase in urine steroid excretion during the long tetracosactrin test is consistent with secondary adrenocortical insufficiency whereas no increase is found in the primary type.

Side-effects   The administration of tetracosactrin depot for three days may very rarely cause sodium and water retention with the risk of oedema, while the marked and prolonged increase in circulating corticosteroid levels that may occur in patients with bilateral adrenal hyperplasia can cause a severe exacerbation of the symptoms of Cushing's syndrome. On extremely rare occasions, adrenal crisis has supervened during prolonged ACTH stimulation in patients with marked adrenal insufficiency. For this reason, some clinicians give 1 mg of dexamethasone daily through the three days on which tetracosactrin depot is given to provide steroid cover. This does not interfere with the test and is regarded as a sensible precaution.

Causes of an abnormal cortisol response to tetracosactrin

Impaired response
1. Cushing's syndrome associated with an adrenal adenoma or carcinoma.
2. Cushing's syndrome due to ectopic ACTH production at a rate sufficient to stimulate the adrenal maximally.
3.   Primary adrenocortical insufficiency.
4. Secondary adrenocortical insufficiency due to:
    (*a*) Prolonged hypothalamic or anterior–pituitary hypofunction
    (*b*) Interruption of the hypothalamic–hypophyseal portal vascular system
    (*c*) Prolonged corticosteroid therapy.

Exaggerated response
1. In some patients with bilateral adrenal hyperplasia due to the over-production of ACTH by the pituitary (Cushing's disease).
2. After the prior administration of ACTH.
3. In some patients with an impaired ability to clear cortisol from the circulation.

Insulin stress test

THIS TEST IS POTENTIALLY DANGEROUS but it is, however, perfectly safe providing there is adequate supervision and patient care.

The insulin stress test is based on stress responsiveness and the integrity of pathways leading to the hypothalmus. A reproducible and standardized stress is used in the form of insulin-induced hypoglycaemia. In normal subjects a fall in blood glucose concentration below 2.2 mmol/ℓ is associated with a marked rise in plasma ACTH and cortisol, with simultaneous increases in growth hormone and catecholamines. It is probably the most sensitive index of hypothalamic or pituitary dysfunction and is of considerable value in the investigation of secondary adrenocortical insufficiency.

Patient care
Before the test:
Patient care before the test must include the following procedures:

1. Check drugs for interference.
2. ECG – ischaemic changes or history of angina are a contra-indication to the test.
3. The weight of the patient must be measured on the day before test.
4. Exclude both hypothyroidism and severe adrenal insufficiency, or place the patient on the appropriate therapy during the test.
5. Fasting blood sugar should be below 8.3 mmol/ℓ. With diabetics, special management before the test may be necessary to achieve this.
6. Patients must fast from midnight preceding the day of the test and be at rest in bed.

During the test:
A DOCTOR MUST BE PRESENT THROUGHOUT THE TEST and have available at the bedside:

1. Sterile 50% glucose solution for intravenous injection.
2. Glucagon, 0.5 to 1.0 mg.

The presence and duration of hypoglycaemic symptoms, and the insulin dose must be recorded on the laboratory request form. If the patient develops angina, becomes shocked or cannot answer simple questions, intravenous glucose must be given and sampling from a different vein continued. If the patient remains unconscious intramuscular glucagon must be given.

The patient should usually sweat when hypoglycaemic. Sweating is usually mild and only lasts for 10 to 15 minutes.

After the test:

1. Give a 20 g glucose drink followed by breakfast; 5 mg prednisone should be added to the drink if it is suspected that the patient has hypopituitarism.
2. Ensure that the patient has a meal every four hours for the remainder of the day.

Method   The dosage of soluble insulin should be as follows:
Standard – 0.10 units/kg in suspected hypopituitarism, 0.15 units/kg in probable normals;
Augmented – 0.3 units/kg if insulin resistance is expected (for example, obesity, acromegaly, Cushing's syndrome, some diabetics).

Venous blood samples are collected preferably from an indwelling venous cannula, which must be washed out with heparinised saline solution after taking each sample. The heparinised saline solution must always be withdrawn before taking subsequent samples.

Samples to be collected are:
Blood glucose – 1 ml in a fluoride tube.
Cortisol – 5 ml in a heparin or plain tube.
In this test the growth hormone (GH) response can also be measured, and in this case:
Cortisol and GH – full 10 ml in a plain tube.
The actual times of the samples must be recorded on request forms and blood tubes as shown in *Table 3.2*.

Table 3.2

Time (min)	−2	0	+20	+30	+60	+90	+120
Glucose	+	Insulin	+	+	+	+	+
Cortisol	+	Intravenous		+	+	+	+
GH	+			+	+	+	+
(± TSH)	(+)		(+)		(+)		

The TRH test (*see* page 6) and LH–RH test (*see* page 20) can also be done at the same time if indicated. In this situation Relefact (1 ampoule contains 100 µg LH–RH and 200 µg TRH) and insulin are given simultaneously; 5 ml of blood in a plain tube is then also collected at the times shown for TSH.

Normal responses The maximum plasma *cortisol* value should reach 550 nmol/ℓ and the increment on the basal value should exceed 190 nmol/ℓ.

The maximum *growth hormone* value should reach 20 mU/ℓ. Patients with severe GH deficiency have values of less than 7 mU/ℓ throughout, and in those with partial deficiency a peak value of about 15 mU/ℓ is found. Peak values between 15 and 20 mU/ℓ are of doubtful significance.

The insulin stress test is a most valuable procedure, being sensitive and reliable. Failure to obtain an ACTH/cortisol response to hypoglycaemia, accompanied by the subsequent demonstration of a normal ACTH/cortisol response to corticotrophin releasing hormone (CRH) suggests the lesion is at the hypothalamic level rather than at the pituitary level since CRH causes release of any ACTH present in the adenohypophysis, probably by a direct action, whereas the hypoglycaemic response requires an intact hypothalamo-pituitary-adrenal axis.

The test also allows simultaneous assessment of the ability to secrete growth hormone and unlike the metyrapone test it answers the question: Can the patient respond adequately to stress? A normal hypoglycaemic response indicates that the patient will respond adequately to stress and therefore does not require corticosteroid replacement therapy, whereas an impaired response implies the need for replacement. This test is also valuable in corticosteroid-treated patients since it indicates whether corticosteroid cover for surgery will be required.

Causes of an impaired plasma cortisol response to insulin-induced hypoglycaemia

An impaired plasma cortisol response to this test can be caused by the following:

1. Hypothalamic*, anterior pituitary* or adrenocortical hypofunction.

*Many patients with hypothalamic or pituitary dysfunction who maintain a normal corticosteroid response have an impaired or absent rise in circulating growth hormone levels during insulin-induced hypoglycaemia.

2. Interruption of the hypothalamic-hypophyseal portal vascular system.
3. Anorexia nervosa† or severe malnutrition due to some other cause.
4. Cushing's syndrome with the exception of some patients with ectopic ACTH production.
5. Failure to achieve an adequate degree of hypoglycaemia due to:
   (*a*) Failure to inject the correct amount of insulin (which may result from not washing out the syringe fully)
   (*b*) Insulin resistance – as in obesity, Cushing's syndrome or acromegaly
   (*c*) Initial hyperglycaemia (as in diabetes mellitus) or the ingestion of carbohydrate during the test.
6. High initial plasma cortisol value, due to anxiety or leaving insufficient time between inserting an indwelling needle and starting the test. These stressful stimuli may be decreasing at the time hypoglycaemia is inducing a response with the result that plasma cortisol values remain high but do not show the expected increment during the test.

Dexamethasone suppression tests

Full dexamethasone suppression test
Dexamethasone, a potent glucocorticoid, suppresses endogenous ACTH secretion in normal subjects acting through the negative feedback control mechanism. The changes in ACTH are monitored by changes in urine steroids and plasma cortisol, since dexamethasone does not interfere with these measurements.

Method   The patient should not be receiving oestrogens or spironolactone, and preferably on no drugs at all.
   The test schedule covers six days with daily 24-hour urine collections, and blood for cortisol estimation with dexamethasone given over the four days as detailed in *Table 3.3*.

---

†Some patients with anorexia nervosa have high circulating corticosteroid levels which fail to rise in response to hypoglycaemia.

Table 3.3 Full dexamethasone suppression test schedule

Day	Dose	24 h Urine 17-oxogenic steroids or free cortisol[1]	Plasma cortisol 0900h
1	Basal	+	*
2	Basal	+	+
3	Dexamethasone 0.5 mg q.i.d.	+	
4	Dexamethasone 0.5 mg q.i.d.	+	+
5	Dexamethasone 2.0 mg q.i.d.	+	
6	Dexamethasone 2.0 mg q.i.d.	+	+

+ Blood and urine collections.
* Midnight plasma cortisol should also be collected on day 1.
[1] As a routine, only the specimens from days 1, 4 and 6 should be estimated; however, all specimens must be sent to the laboratory.

Normal response   In normal subjects the urine 17-oxogenic steroid excretion should fall to less than 17 μmol/24 hours or free cortisol to less than 69 nmol/24 hours (25 μg/24 hours). In contrast, more than 94% of patients with Cushing's syndrome, irrespective of its cause, show inadequate suppression. The larger dose of dexamethasone is employed to establish the aetiology of the syndrome (*see* the section on Cushing's syndrome on page 41).

Side-effects and problems   This test has a number of disadvantages, foremost among which is that it requires six consecutive 24-hour urine collections which must be done with care to avoid spuriously low results due to their being incomplete; regular administration of dexamethasone is required; urine analysis is relatively difficult and time-consuming; finally, the administration of such large amounts of steroid may cause an exacerbation of the symptoms of Cushing's syndrome and result in complications such as septicaemia. In many patients, therefore, the short dexamethasone suppression test is an attractive alternative certainly as an initial screening procedure.

Short dexamethasone suppression test

The principle of the short test is the same as that of the long test which has already been described.

Method   Day 1 – 0900 hours – blood for basal plasma cortisol is collected. Between 2200 and 2400 hours a single oral dose of 1 mg of dexamethasone is given.
Day 2 – 0900 hours – blood for plasma cortisol is collected.

Normal response   In normal subjects plasma cortisol on day 2 should fall to a value of less than 180 nmol/ℓ, and this should represent a fall of at least 70% below the subject's basal value on day 1. Patients with Cushing's syndrome, irrespective of the aetiology, fail to show normal suppression. The test is of no value in differentiating between the various causes of Cushing's syndrome. It is essentially a rapid screening test which if positive warrants proceeding to the full dexamethasone suppression test. Failure to suppress may occur in obesity and in patients on phenytoin and oestrogens.

Metyrapone test

Metyrapone (Metopirone) inhibits (among other enzyme systems) 11β-hydroxylase which is involved in the final step of cortisol synthesis. The consequent fall in plasma cortisol stimulates ACTH secretion via the feedback mechanism which accelerates steroid biosynthesis. As a result 11-deoxycortisol, the immediate precursor of cortisol, is released into the circulation and is then metabolized by the liver, mainly to its tetrahydro derivative, and excreted in the urine. The test is based on the fact that 11-deoxycortisol, unlike cortisol, does not suppress ACTH secretion. The metabolites of 11-deoxycortisol can be determined in the urine as 17-oxogenic steroids.

Method   The patient should not be receiving any drugs liable to interfere with the urine steroid assay.

Table 3.4 Metyrapone test

Day	Dose	24h Urine 17-oxogenic steroids
1	Basal	+
2	Metyrapone 750 mg 4 hourly × 6	+
3	Metyrapone 750 mg 4 hourly × 6	+

As a routine only the specimens from days 1 and 3 will be estimated; however, all specimens should be sent to the laboratory.

Normal response An increment of at least 35 μmol/24 hours in urine 17-oxogenic steroids on day 3 when compared with the basal value on day 1.

Side-effects and precautions The patient should be warned that he may experience slight nausea and dizziness in the period following administration of each dose of metyrapone. This side-effect will be lessened if the drug is taken with some milk.

Because of the enzyme inhibitory effect of the drug it should *not* be administered during pregnancy.

Diagnostic considerations

Adrenocortical hyperplasia (Cushing's syndrome)

Cushing's syndrome results from sustained and inappropriately raised plasma free cortisol concentrations. The characteristic features are central obesity, a plethoric moon face, hypertension, purple striae, osteoporosis, muscular weakness and wasting, hyperglycaemia and mental changes. In women hirsutism and menstrual disturbances are common.

The management of the patient with Cushing's syndrome is two-fold. First the diagnosis must be established and, secondly, the cause must be found. The treatment will vary depending on the aetiology.

The causes of Cushing's syndrome are:

1. ACTH. dependent causes:
   (*a*) pituitary tumour
   (*b*) increased CRF production
   (*c*) ectopic ACTH syndrome
   (*d*) iatrogenic
2. Non-ACTH. dependent:
   (*a*) adrenal adenoma or carcinoma
   (*b*) iatrogenic

The most reliable investigations to establish the diagnosis of Cushing's syndrome are as follows:

1. *Abolition of the normal nyctohemeral variation.* This occurs in plasma cortisol due to elevation of the midnight level. The rhythm is abolished in nearly every patient with Cushing's syndrome. It is also abolished in many acutely ill patients, in some alcoholics and in 50% of patients with depression.
2. *Raised urinary cortisol.* The 24 hourly urinary cortisol is more specific than the 17-hydroxycorticosteroid. It is raised in over 95% of patients with Cushing's syndrome. It is also raised in many acutely ill medical patients, a majority of post-operative patients and virtually all pregnant women.
3. *Overnight dexamethasone suppression test.* In over 99% of patients with Cushing's syndrome there is a failure to suppress the 0900 hours plasma cortisol following dexamethasone 1 mg at 2300 hours the previous night. A few obese patients fail to suppress and also a significant proportion who are chronically ill, depressed or alcoholic. This group of patients will, however, have a normal insulin tolerance test.

The most useful investigations to determine the causes of Cushing's syndrome are:

1. *Plasma ACTH level.* This is undetectable in patients with adrenal tumours. It is raised in ACTH dependent causes. Extremely high levels tend to occur in ectopic ACTH syndromes, but there is considerable overlap with patients with pituitary dependent Cushing's syndrome in the 100–200 pg/ml range.
2. *High dose dexamethasone suppression.* In 98% of patients with pituitary dependent Cushing's syndrome the urinary oxogenic and urinary cortisol excretion is suppressed. Six per cent of patients with the ectopic ACTH syndrome will suppress but this is not the case in patients with adrenal tumours.

It is sometimes extremely difficult to segregate patients with pituitary dependent Cushing's syndrome from patients with ectopic ACTH syndrome. In difficult cases it may be necessary to undertake selective venous sampling of the internal jugular vein to confirm pituitary dependent disease. It is also advisable to have a

CT scan of the chest and abdomen to exclude bronchial carcinoids and tumours of the pancreas.

Adrenocortical hypofunction

Adrenocortical hypofunction may be either primary (Addison's disease) or secondary to a failure of ACTH production caused either by hypothalamic-pituitary disease, or from suppression following treatment with pharmacological doses of steroids.

The clinical features of primary adrenal hypofunction are tiredness, anorexia and nausea, pigmentation, vomiting, weight loss and hypotension. In secondary adrenocortical hypofunction due to hypothalamic-pituitary disease these may also be associated with the features of hypopituitarism (*see* page 23). In primary adrenal insufficiency there is often an increase in plasma potassium and urea with a fall in sodium due to decreased aldosterone production.

The diagnostic biochemical features are:

1. Abolition of the normal nyctohemeral variation in plasma cortisol due to low 0900 hours value.
2. Failure of response in plasma cortisol to tetracosactrin.
3. Differentiation between primary and secondary adrenal hypofunction can be done by measurement of plasma ACTH concentration which is high in primary and low in secondary stages.

Note: Plasma cortisol may be low in primary hypothyroidism.

4 Hypothalamic–posterior pituitary disorders

Physiology

The posterior pituitary hormones *vasopressin* (antidiuretic hormone (ADH)) and *oxytocin* are synthesized in the cells of the anterior hypothalamic nuclei and then pass down the pituitary stalk along the axonal nerve fibres which run from those cells. The axonal fibres terminate in the posterior lobe of the pituitary. The hormones are stored in granules in the terminal bulbs of the axonal fibres and are secreted directly into the bloodstream in response to neurogenic stimuli.

Vasopressin and oxytocin are similar in structure and each consists of a peptide containing only eight amino acid residues. They are synthesized, stored and secreted with a larger protein, *neurophysin*, which is of uncertain function, but which binds the smaller peptides and may act as a storage molecule.

Vasopressin secretion occurs in response to three major stimulatory mechanisms, as follows:

1. An increase in plasma osmotic pressure, a mechanism which involves osmoreceptors located in the anterior hypothalamic nuclei.
2. A decrease in plasma volume, involving volume receptors which are located in the major central veins and the onward transmission of impulses to the paraventricular and supra-optic nuclei.

3. Physical or psychological stresses, acting through 'higher' centres in the brain with their final common pathway through the paraventricular and supra-optic nuclei. Drugs may also be included under this heading; some stimulate while others inhibit vasopressin secretion. Stimulators include barbiturates and narcotics, including anaesthesia. Inhibitors include ethanol and diphenylhydantoin.

Vasopressin is the single and most important hormonal factor in the regulation of renal water excretion and the production of concentrated urine. The action of vasopressin involves cyclic 3',5'-AMP with a consequent alteration in water permeability of the distal renal tubules and collecting ducts. The renal handling of water is intimately linked with sodium and the factors which enhance the secretion of vasopressin also affect aldosterone secretion rate either directly or indirectly through the renin-angiotensin system.

Oxytocin secretion appears to be stimulated by receptors in the breast (the 'suckling' reflex) and the uterus. The hormone action on both of those organs is dependent on previous 'conditioning' by ovarian and placental hormones during pregnancy. The action of oxytocin on the uterus is to cause smooth muscle contraction with a maximum effect at term and during labour. On the breast, oxytocin causes contraction of the myoepithelial cells which results in milk being squeezed from the alveoli and finer ducts into the larger systems leading to the nipple, with consequent 'milk ejection'.

Specimens and normal range values

Assays have been developed for these two hormones but are *not available* as routine procedures.

The concentration of oxytocin in peripheral venous blood from adults is generally undetectable, even during pregnancy, and becomes measurable only with the onset of labour. There are no clinical indications for the estimation of oxytocin, as there are no known diseases caused by either an excess or deficiency of this hormone.

The assay of plasma vasopressin is technically difficult because of the very low circulating peripheral venous blood concentrations. Urine vasopressin estimation is only of limited value potentially in differentiating between the two types of diabetes insipidus or in the diagnosis of 'inappropriate' ADH secretion. Urine samples for vasopressin estimation must be collected under strictly defined conditions as the secretion of this hormone is dependent on both plasma volume and osmolality; it is also affected by a wide range of drugs. As the differentiation between the two forms of diabetes insipidus and the diagnosis of inappropriate ADH secretion can be established by osmometry, the urine vasopressin assay is only necessary in exceptional circumstances.

Diagnostic considerations

Diabetes insipidus

Diabetes insipidus is a rare disease in which there is inability to concentrate urine.

A clinical feature of this disease is that a large volume of dilute urine is passed throughout the 24-hour cycle. There is normally a circadian or nyctohemeral decrease in the urine secretion rate at night with a simultaneous reduction in volume and increase in concentration. This is thought to be due mainly to nyctohemeral rhythm of vasopressin secretion in addition to other factors such as changes in renal blood flow and glomerular filtration rate (GFR) during sleep.

The causes of diabetes insipidus are either a lack of vasopressin (*cranial diabetes insipidus*) or resistance/insensitivity at the target site (*nephrogenic diabetes insipidus*). These conditions can be confused with patients who are 'compulsive water drinkers' – a psychiatric disturbance in which thirst is the dominant feature. In these patients, although plasma and urine osmolality may be low, the renal tubules retain the ability to concentrate urine in response to the challenge of water deprivation. If, however, their disturbance has been of a long duration they may occasionally have a minor degree of impairment in urine concentrating ability.

Cranial diabetes insipidus

Cranial diabetes insipidus, with a lack of vasopressin, may be caused by the following conditions:

1. Pituitary or hypothalamic tumours: adenoma, craniopharyngioma, suprasellar meningioma or a glioma, metastatic lesions (particularly from the breast or lung).
2. Infections or granulomas: tuberculous basal meningitis, sarcoidosis, encephalitis, histiocytosis-X.
3. Vascular lesions.
4. Trauma, surgery or radiation.
5. Idiopathic or familial, either dominant or recessive, and may be associated with diabetes mellitus.

Many of these are conditions that cause hypopituitarism due to anterior lobe hormone deficiency (*see* page 23), and anterior pituitary function should also be investigated in these patients.

Nephrogenic diabetes insipidus

Nephrogenic diabetes insipidus, with target organ resistance to vasopressin, may be either acquired or congenital. The latter is a rare sex-linked disorder, usually recessive, showing a variable degree of penetrance in female heterozygotes. The symptom of polyuria usually appears soon after birth in male infants and because of their excessive drinking there may be an associated growth failure, the consequence of inadequate eating. The acquired form may occur in patients with chronic renal failure, hypokalaemia, hypercalcaemia, lithium toxicity, after renal transplant, tubular lesions (myeloma, amyloidosis and Sjögren's syndrome) and sickle cell anaemia.

Water deprivation test

This test should only be undertaken in adequately hydrated patients, and only then with careful and continuous supervision. Patients with severe diabetes insipidus may become extremely dehydrated (primary water depletion) with consequent circulatory failure, while 'compulsive water drinkers' may cheat!

The basis of this test is the comparison and measurement of plasma and urine osmolalities during eight hours of fluid deprivation, followed by the effect of exogenous vasopressin on these two variables.

Patient care   Patient care before and during the test should consist of the following:

1. *No* previous overnight fluid restriction.
2. Prior to the commencement of the test the patient may have a light breakfast but *no* tea or coffee.
3. Smoking is not permitted throughout the test period.
4. The patient should be weighed immediately prior to the commencement of the test, and then at two-hour intervals throughout; *the test should be stopped* if there is loss of more than 5% of initial body weight, and/or if the patient becomes shocked.
5. *No* fluids are allowed once the test period has commenced.
6. If the patient is already receiving desmopressin treatment this should be stopped for 24 hours.
7. *No* alcohol.

Method   The test should be conducted as follows:

1. At 0800 hours, urine is passed and the specimen is discarded.
2. Samples to be collected:
    (*a*) Venous blood samples preferably from an indwelling catheter – 5 ml in heparin tube
    (*b*) Urine into clean containers

Blood and urine samples must be taken to the laboratory for the measurement of osmolality as soon as possible after collection.

Urine collections are made on an hourly basis with blood samples in the middle of some of the collection periods as shown in *Table 4.1*.

Vasopressin may be given as desmopressin (DDAVP), 20 µg intranasally. The advantages of this synthetic analogue is that unlike other forms of vasopressin it does not possess any pressor activity, nor does it cause smooth muscle contraction; its use, therefore, avoids any untoward side-effects (pallor, colic, bronchospasm, coronary artery or uterine spasm).

Table 4.1

Urine	Blood
0800–0900h Urine 1*	0830h Blood 1
0900–1000h Urine 2	
1000–1100h Urine 3	
1100–1200h Urine 4*	1130h Blood 2
1200–1300h Urine 5	
1300–1400h Urine 6	
1400–1500h Urine 7*	1430h Blood 3
1500–1600h Urine 8*	1530h Blood 4
1601h Give vasopressin	
1600–1700h Urine 9*	
1700–1800h Urine 10*	1730h Blood 5
1800–1900h Urine 11*	1930h Blood 6
1900–2000h Urine 12*	

All of the blood samples (1–6) and the marked* urine samples (1, 4, 7–12) have their osmolality measured, and all of the urine specimens must have their volume recorded.

Interpretation   In the normal response the plasma osmolality should not exceed 300m osmol/kg while the urine value should reach more than 600m osmol/kg with a ratio of more than 1.9 for the osmolalities of urine 7/blood 3 and urine 8/blood 4.

In patients with cranial diabetes insipidus, because of the lack of vasopressin and consequent water loss, the plasma osmolality increases to more than 300m osmol/kg while the urine value remains low with ratios of less than 1.9 for the osmolalities of urine 7/blood 3 and urine 8/blood 4. After the administration of vasopressin to these patients there should be a normal response with urine concentration and a fall in plasma osmolality.

Patients with nephrogenic diabetes insipidus will show an initial response which will be comparable to that in patients with primary lack of vasopressin but with a failure to concentrate after the administration of vasopressin.

Compulsive water drinkers should have a normal response pattern to water deprivation and should *not* go on to a vasopressin test in view of the danger of water intoxication. It is usually possible to differentiate patients with compulsive water drinking from those with diabetes insipidus by measurement of serum osmolality. In the former group osmolality is low while it is increased in patients with diabetes insipidus.

'Inappropriate' ADH syndrome

The inappropriate secretion of vasopressin (ADH) is recognized to occur in a number of situations. The resultant syndrome is due to excessive water retention which persists despite a concomitant reduction in plasma osmolality.

Clinically, if the plasma sodium concentration does not fall below 120 nmol/ℓ the patient may be asymptomatic. At lower plasma sodium concentrations the clinical features are those of water intoxication, initially with anorexia followed by nausea and vomiting, also irritability with personality changes of unco-operation and confusion. At a plasma sodium concentration of less than 110 mmol/ℓ marked neurological abnormalities may occur – a decrease or loss of reflexes, muscle weakness, bulbar palsy – progressing to stupor with or without convulsive episodes.

The principal causes of this syndrome are:

1. Malignant tumours: carcinoma of lung (oat cell type); carcinoma of duodenum; carcinoma of pancreas; thymoma.
2. Disorders of the central nervous system: meningitis; head injuries; abscess; tumours; encephalitis; Guillain-Barré syndrome; subarachnoid haemorrhage; acute intermittent porphyria.
3. Pulmonary diseases: pneumonia; tuberculosis; cavitation (aspergillosis), prolonged mechanical ventilation.
4. Idiopathic.

It is also possible that the inappropriate secretion of vasopressin may play a role in the development of hyponatraemia and water retention in patients with: endocrine disorders such as Addison's disease, myxoedema, hypopituitarism; the immediate post-operative period; cardiac failure; cirrhosis of the liver.

In these situations the term 'inappropriate' may be incorrect in that ADH may be appropriately secreted for a lower osmostat setting or that hyponatraemia may be due to causes other than excessive ADH secretion.

The essential findings of this syndrome are:

1. Hyponatraemia with hypo-osmolality of plasma.
2. Continued renal excretion of sodium despite hyponatraemia.

3. Urine osmolality which is greater than expected when considered in relationship to the concomitant plasma osmolality;
   that is, the urine is less than maximally dilute.
4. Absence of clinical evidence of fluid volume depletion.
5. Normal renal function.
6. Normal adrenal function.

The diagnosis of this syndrome is dependent, therefore, on the
presence of the above findings, the most critical of which is that
the urine is less than maximally dilute.

5 Adrenal cortical disorders

Physiology

The adrenal cortex secretes three main groups of hormones –
glucocorticoids, *mineralocorticoids* and *androgens* (*see Figure 5.1*).
It also produces other steroids some of which, for example,
progesterone, have a biological activity and can be measured as
plasma 17-α-hydroxyprogesterone.

The main glucocorticoid is *cortisol* although some *corticosterone*
is also produced. The secretion rate of these corticosteroids is
under the influence of the adrenocorticotrophic hormone (ACTH)
(*see* page 29).

Aldosterone, which is produced in the zona glomerulosa of the
adrenal cortex, is the most important of the mineralocorticoids;
others include deoxycorticosterone and 17-OH deoxycorticosterone but these are only normally produced in small amounts. The
adrenal secretion rate of aldosterone is largely independent of
ACTH and is controlled by sodium status indirectly through the
renin-angiotensin system; *potassium* ion also has a direct effect on
secretion rate. The renal juxtaglomerular cells in response to
variations in renal perfusion pressure (which is directly related to
circulating blood volume and sodium status) release renin. The
latter, an enzyme, acts on a circulating globulin *angiotensinogen*
with the formation of the decapeptide *angiotensin I*. The latter is
subsequently converted in the lungs to the octapeptide *angiotensin
II*. Angiotensin II not only stimulates aldosterone production but
is also a potent pressor substance. Aldosterone affects the distal

52

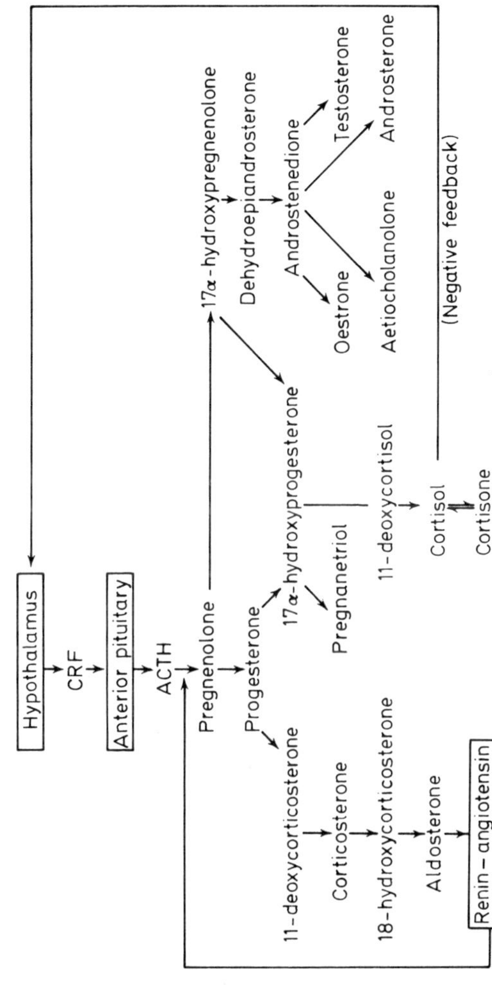

Figure 5.1 Hormones of the adrenal cortex

renal tubular handling of sodium; renal sodium retention causes an increase in total body sodium, with a consequent increase in total body water, extracellular and plasma volume.

The *adrenal androgens* are relatively weak androgenic compounds when compared with testosterone. In adults they are produced in large amounts by the adrenal cortex in both males and females. Prior to puberty their secretion rate is low and then increases at that time to adult values – probably playing an important part in the growth spurt of puberty. Their secretion at this stage appears to be regulated by ACTH.

Specimens and normal range values

Plasma cortisol (see page 30)

The following assays can only be undertaken after special previous arrangements with the laboratory.

Plasma renin and aldosterone

The secretion rates of both renin and aldosterone vary with the time of the day, posture, emotional stress and drug therapy and salt status. It is *essential*, therefore, that when samples are collected the patients should be under standardized conditions.

Blood for either of these assays (10 ml of venous blood into a pre-cooled herparin tube for plasma aldosterone and 5 ml in a pre-cooled Na-EDTa tube for plasma renin activity) should be collected between 0800 and 0900 hours with the patient still recumbent in bed from the previous night's sleep (a minimum of eight hours in the horizontal position!). In the case of renin a second sample should also be collected 30 minutes later during which time the patient has been either standing or walking quietly. The samples must be kept surrounded with ice and taken to the laboratory *immediately* after collection.

As a number of drugs (hypotensives, diuretics, purgatives and contraceptives, etc.) affect the renin-angiotensin system, all medication should be discontinued for at least three weeks prior to the assay of renin and aldosterone. The latter is also affected by electrolyte status and for at least the three days prior to aldosterone sample collection the patient should receive a minimum daily intake of 100 mmol of sodium and between 50 and 70 mmol of potassium.

Plasma 17-α-hydroxyprogesterone

1. The child should be aged more than 48 hours.
2. As this compound shows a marked circadian or nyctohemeral variation blood should be collected when potentially at maximum values between 0800 and 0900 hours.
3. Blood should be taken prior to the commencement of any steroid medication.
4. Venous blood (1 ml) in a paediatric lithium container should be taken immediately to the laboratory for separation and storage at 4°C; *not* frozen.

Urine pregnanetriol

1. No particular patient preparation is required for this test.
2. A complete 24-hour urine sample is collected into a container, to which has been added 10 ml of 2% boric acid as a preservative.

The normal range values are:
Under 6 years of age – Mean 0.6 μmol/24 hours
6 to 16 years – 1.0 to 3.5 μmol/24 hours
Over 16 years – 1.0 to 10.5 μmol/24 hours

Urine 11-oxygenation index

The 11-oxygenation index (non-11-oxygenated 17-oxogenic steroids divided by 11-oxygenated 17-oxogenic steroids) reflects the efficiency of the last stages of the biosynthesis of cortisol. It is of value in the biochemical confirmation of the clinical diagnosis of congenital adrenal hyperplasia.

1. The patient should be aged more than 8 days.
2. No particular preparation of the patient is required, but the sample should be collected prior to treatment with steroids.

3. A random clean sample of urine is collected, with a minimum
   volume of 10 ml, to which is added a few drops of 2% boric acid
   as a preservative. The normal ratio is less than 0.7.

Diagnostic considerations

Adrenocortical disorders may be classified as follows:

1. Hypofunction: primary; secondary – hypopituitarism, steroid
   therapy.
2. Hyperfunction – Cushing's syndrome (*see* page 41).
3. Congenital adrenal hyperplasia.
4. Hyperaldosteronism: primary; secondary.
5. Hypoaldosteronism.

Primary adrenocortical hypofunction (Addison's disease)

Addison's disease, when originally described, was mainly due to
tuberculous destruction of the adrenal glands; the most common
cause now (approximately 60% of cases) is atrophy of the cortices
(an autoimmune process), with the remainder due to carcinoma-
tosis (either metastatic deposits or therapeutic removal), amyloidosis, tuberculosis and fungal infections. Addison's disease may
also occur acutely from bilateral haemorrhages into the adrenal
glands.

The clinical features (*see* page 43) are mainly due to the
deficiency of both glucocorticoids and mineralocorticoids. The
pigmentation is due to overproduction of ACTH as the result of
low cortisol feedback.

For the diagnostic biochemical features, *see* page 43.

Secondary adrenocortical hypofunction

Secondary hypofunction may occur as a feature of hypopituitarism
(*see* page 23).

The commonest cause of hypoadrenalism is suppression of the
hypothalamic–pituitary–adrenocortical axis by long-term corticos-

teroid therapy. The risk of suppression is related to both the dose and the duration of steroid therpay.

A daily dose of, or exceeding, 40 mg of cortisol or its equivalent can cause suppression, a smaller dose may do so if given over a long period. The comparative potencies of different glucocorticoids are shown in *Table 5.1*.

Table 5.1

Glucocorticoid	Equivalent doses (mg)
Cortisol	25
Cortisone	20
Prednisone	5
Prednisolone	5
Methyl prednisolone	4
Triamcinolone	4
Betamethasone	0.75
Dexamethasone	0.75

The clinical features of secondary adrenocortical hypofunction are given on page 43.

The diagnostic biochemical features are as in primary failure, but in the secondary situation there is a reduction in ACTH secretion.

Congenital adrenal hyperplasia

This disease is a result of inherited inborn defects in the hydroxylating enzymes of the adrenal gland which normally convert progesterone into hydrocortisone, corticosterone and aldosterone. The defects, of which there are several, result in the accumulation of androgenic precursors which cause virilization, accelerated growth and epiphyseal ossification. As the secretion of the adrenal androgens is controlled by ACTH the enhanced pituitary stimulation, which arises because of the low serum levels of hydrocortisone, further increases androgen production. Two hydroxylations are involved in the synthesis of hydrocortisone from 17-hydroxyprogesterone and each requires a specific enzyme. The more important varieties of congenital hyperplasia result from defects of the 21-hydroxylase and 11-hydroxylase enzymes.

Progesterone

> Hydroxylation
> at C17

17 - hydroxyprogesterone

> Hydroxylation
> at C21

11 - deoxyhydrocortisone (Compound S)

> Hydroxylation
> at C11

Hydrocortisone

A third less common type has been described in which a block occurs, preventing the formation of progesterone.

If there is a partial block of the 21-hydroxylase system the plasma hydrocortisone level may be maintained by the increased secretion of ACTH. However, despite the increase in ACTH, the hydrocortisone level may be below normal and children with this defect are unlikely to be able to survive stress. They are also liable to salt loss as there is in addition an abnormality in the synthesis of aldosterone. Lack of the enzyme 11-hydroxylase stops synthesis of hydrocortisone at the stage of compound S and also prevents the formation of corticosterone from 11-deoxycorticosterone. The accumulation of deoxycorticosterone leads to hypertension and the inability to form hydrocortisone to adrenal insufficiency.

Progressive virilization is the most conspicuous manifestation of this disease and is due to the excessive production of androgens. The rapid growth, increased musculature and accelerated epiphyseal growth are due to the protein anabolic action of the androgen. In the female virilization of the external genitalia takes place and the infant is readily mistaken for a male with undescended testes.

The biochemical diagnosis is initially based on the estimation of urinary 17-oxogenic steroids. However, in the neonatal period raised levels are not always seen and rapid changes in excretion of these steroids makes interpretation of the results difficult.

In 21-hydroxylase deficiency there is an increase in 17-hydroxyprogesterone with a consequent increase in circulating plasma values and in the urinary metabolite pregnanetriol. The urinary 11-oxygenation index (the ratio of 11-deoxy to 11-oxy fractions) in normal children is less than 0.7 and can be markedly increased in severe 21-hydroxylase deficiency. These abnormalities are rapidly corrected by the administration of physiological amounts of cortisol.

Primary hyperaldosteronism (Conn's syndrome)

This condition may be defined as autonomous hypersecretion of aldosterone by the adrenal gland. In approximately two-thirds of cases this is due to a discrete unilateral adenoma, while in the remainder it is due to bilateral hyperplasia. The excess of aldosterone results in renal sodium retention, an increased total body sodium with an increase in plasma volume and hypertension. These changes are usually associated with urinary potassium loss and hypokalaemia, although some normokalaemic cases have been reported.

The clinical features of the syndrome are hypertension in association with muscular weakness, polyuria and headaches. The muscle weakness may vary from a slight impairment to attacks of paralysis.

The diagnostic biochemical features include a hypokalaemic metabolic alkalosis, high plasma sodium, low plasma renin with an increased aldosterone. However, low renin values occur in approximately 20% of patients with essential hypertension and an increase in aldosterone can be secondary to other conditions. A definitive procedure is therefore to repeat the assay of these two after either sodium loading or mineralocorticoid suppressive therapy (*see* also screening procedures below). In approximately half of the cases there is an impairment in glucose tolerance as a consequence of hypokalaemia-induced defective insulin release. Other causes of hypokalaemia must always be excluded. These include:

1. Treatment with diuretics.
2. Excessive use of purgatives.
3. Vomiting.
4. Excessive intake of either liquorice or carbenoxolone (these contain glycyrrhetinic acid, or a derivative, and this has an aldosterone-like action).
5. Renal tubular potassium 'leak' (Liddle's disease).

In view of the problems of availability of aldosterone and renin assays a variety of simple screening procedures have been proposed which measure hormonal effect rather than concentration. The most useful of which is sodium loading – a normal plasma potassium concentration should be maintained in hypertensive patients (who do not have evidence of either renal disease, coarctation of the aorta or phaeochromocytoma) after 14 days on a high sodium diet (between 150 and 200 mmol/day).

Secondary hyperaldosteronism

This condition may be defined as an increase in aldosterone secretion secondary to an increase in renin. Secondary hyperaldosteronism may be due to:

1. Diuretic (usually of the benzothiadizine group) treatment in hypertension.
2. Renal artery stenosis.
3. Chronic renal disease.
4. Cirrhosis of the liver.
5. The nephrotic syndrome.
6. Congestive cardiac failure.
7. Malignant hypertension.
8. Renin-secreting tumour.
9. Bartter's syndrome – hyperplasia of the juxtaglomerular apparatus, hypokalaemic alkalosis, and aldosteronism with normal blood pressure.

Hypoaldosteronism

Hypoaldosteronism is a rare but potential cause of unexpected hyperkalaemia in the presence of only moderately impaired renal function, usually occurring in old patients.

6 Disorders of the adrenal medulla

Physiology

The adrenal medulla secretes the catecholamines *adrenaline* (epinephrine) and *noradrenaline* (norepinephrine); approximately 80% of production is as adrenaline while 20% is as noradrenaline. Adrenaline is almost exclusively produced by the adrenal medulla and only small amounts are released in the other tissues of the sympathetic nervous system; noradrenaline is produced in sympathetic nerve endings.

The metabolic disposal of catecholamines and their excretion from the body in the urine takes place after catechol-*O*-methylation and oxidative deamination. Adrenaline and noradrenaline undergo *O*-methylation with the formation of *metadrenaline* (metanephrine) and *normetadrenaline* (normetanephrine) respectively. The process of oxidative deamination results in the formation of *3,4-dihydroxymandelic acid* (DHMA) which then undergoes *O*-methylation with the formation of *3-methoxy-4-hydroxymandelic acid*.

The adrenal medulla is *not* essential for the maintenance of life, and interest clincially in the functional status of the gland is limited to hyperfunction and not to hypofunction.

Specimens and normal range values

Plasma

Assays of adrenaline and noradrenaline are *not* available as a routine service, but essentially only a research basis. If blood is to be collected for these assays it is essential that the patient should be prepared in the following manner:

1. The patient should not be stressed, preferably relaxed in bed, and blood sampling should be taken through an indwelling catheter.
2. There should be no drug therapy for at least three days, particularly antihypertensives (especially methyldopa).
3. No coffee or tea should be allowed during or immediately before the sampling period.
4. Specimens should be taken immediately to the laboratory for separation and storage, deep frozen.

Urine

Urinary assays for the diagnosis of adrenal medullary hyperfunction include:

1. VMA (vanilmandelic acid, also known as 3-methoxy-4-hydroxymandelic acid (HMMA)).
2. Total catecholamines.
3. The 3-Methoxy metabolites: metadrenaline, normetadrenaline (neither of these assays are available as a routine service).

The following criteria should be adopted:

1. During the urine collection period (24 hours) and for the preceding 48 hours the patient *should not* consume bananas, citrus fruits, chocolate or foods containing vanilla flavouring, coffee or tea.
2. *All* drug therapy should be stopped, if possible, for at least 48 hours prior to the collection period, particularly antihypertensives (especially methyldopa), phenothiazines, tetracyclines, vitamin preparations and monoamine oxidase inhibitors.
3. The patient should not be stressed during the collection period as this will cause a physiological increase in catecholamines; similarly high values may be found in patients who are either 'ill' or malnourished.

A complete 24-hour urine collection is made into a container to which has been added 15 ml of 6N hydrochloric acid; the pH *must* be maintained at less than 3.

Normal ranges:

HMMA (VMA) 10 to 35 µmol/24 hours.

Total catecholamines less than 600 nmol/24 hours.

Diagnostic considerations

Phaeochromocytoma

Phaeochromocytomas are tumours of chromaffin tissue, occurring in either sex, usually in adults aged 25–55 years, which cause hypertension by their secretion of an excess of catecholamines. The tumours are usually benign. Approximately 90% occur in the adrenal medulla, with the remainder in a variety of intra-abdominal sites, the thorax and the neck. A familial incidence has been reported in association with neurofibromatosis, medullary carcinoma of the thyroid and parathyroid hyperplasia or adenoma.

Phaeochromocytomas account for less than 1% of the hypertensive population but are important because the hypertension is surgically curable. The hypertension may be sustained or paroxysmal depending on whether the tumour's secretion is sustained or occurring in paroxysms. One of the most common symptoms is sweating and the second is palpitations.

The clinical features in a hypertensive patient which warrant further investigation for a phaeochromocytoma are attributable to the paroxysmal secretion of excessive amounts of adrenaline and noradrenaline. The paroxysms can be of a variable duration, lasting from a few minutes to a few hours, and may be precipitated by exercise, local pressure (stooping or straining) or eating citrus fruits (the latter contain an aromatic amine that stimulates the release of adrenaline). The attacks are often preceded by an aura. During the attack there is a marked increase in blood pressure, a throbbing headache, palpitations, pallor and sweating, anxiety and substernal or upper abdominal pain. Some patients have an impairment of glucose tolerance between attacks if the tumour has been present over a long period.

The diagnostic biochemical features are the demonstration of an excessive urinary excretion of catecholamine metabolites either in a random 24-hour sample in patients with persistent hypertension, or in an immediate 'during' and 'post-attack' 24-hour urine collection in patients who are subject to paroxysms. A number of provocative *in vivo* pharmacological tests have been proposed for the investigation of patients with sporadic hypertension using either intravenous histamine or tyramine. These procedures are potentially dangerous and should be avoided.

7 Ovarian disorders

Physiology

The functions of the ovary may be classified under two major headings – gametogenesis, and the secretion of oestrogens.

Gametogenesis

Two successive meiotic divisions precede the formation of the ovum. The first of these reduction divisions (meiosis I) reduces the chromosome number from the diploid (46) to the haploid (23) numbers. The second division (meiosis II) resembles a mitotic division in that each chromosome divides into two chromatids, but the latter are not genetically identical owing to the interchange of genetic material that takes place between homologous chromatids when they come together. In the female all of the primary oocytes have entered the pairing stage of meiosis I by the fifth month of fetal life. At birth, therefore, the ovary of the female child, with approximately half a million follicles, has completed to all intents and purposes its formation of potential ova. The chromosomes remain paired until the ovum is about to be shed at ovulation and the final stage of the first division takes place immediately prior to this event. The second meiotic division takes place after penetration of the ovum by the fertilizing spermatozoa.

During the female reproductive life, an ovum develops as follicular maturation takes place. The expulsion of the ovum from the follicle (ovulation) takes place in the middle of the menstrual cycle and is linked with a number of hormonal changes. The menstrual cycle is divided into the follicular (pre-ovulatory) and luteal (post-ovulatory) phases.

Secretion of oestrogens

The secretions of the ovarian hormones *oestradiol*, *oestrone* and *progesterone* are controlled by the pituitary gonadotrophins FSH and LH. The secretion rates of both FSH and LH are under oestrogen feedback control, while progesterone only influences the secretion of LH. The ovary also secretes small quantities of *androgens* which are normally insignificant but in ovarian disorders can assume clinical importance. The main androgen secreted by the ovary is *androstenedione* and from this is produced approximately two-thirds of the normal female's circulating *testosterone*.

Prepuberty

In the normal child the hypothalamic–pituitary–gonadal axis, although present, is functional only at a very low level. The plasma concentrations of FSH and LH, although measurable, are at low concentrations, with undetectable concentrations of oestradiol. With the advent of puberty there is a steady increase in FSH and LH production which stimulates the ovary to secrete increasing amounts of oestradiol. It is the latter that is responsible to a great extent for the developmental changes that take place over the three to four years of pubertal development – skeletal growth, development of secondary sexual characteristics – and culminate in the onset of menstruation (menarche). Spontaneous regular ovulation only occurs when the hypothalamic–pituitary–ovarian axis is fully developed and does not necessarily coincide with the menarche; there is usually a high incidence of anovulatory cycles around the menarche.

Menstrual cycle (see Figure 7.1)

The follicular phase of the cycle begins with the onset of menstruation. At this time, the pituitary begins to produce low tonic amounts of FSH which in synergy with LH stimulates the maturation of approximately 5–20 follicles per cycle. This is associated

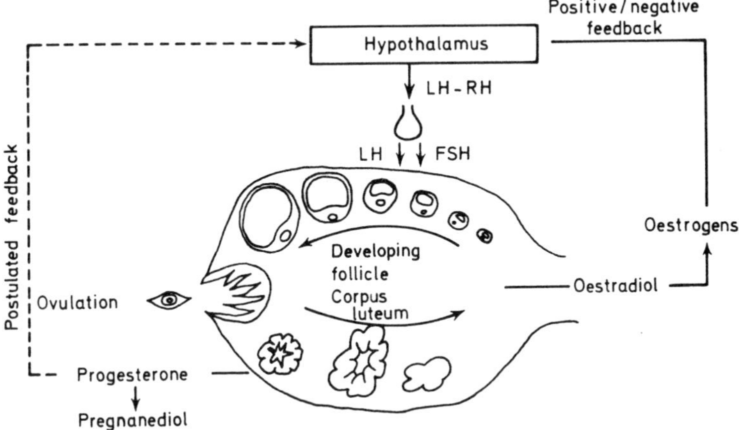

Figure 7.1 Ovarian hormones

with a modest increase in the ovarian secretion of oestradiol. At the mid-follicular phase (day 7–8) nearly all the follicles undergo atresia except the one or two destined to ovulate, which grow exponentially and start secreting significant amounts of oestradiol. The plasma oestradiol concentration increases rapidly and reaches a sharp peak shortly before ovulation. The pre-ovulatory increase of oestrogen and of the associated precursor steroid *17-α-hydroxyprogesterone* are probably secreted by the theca interna cells of the developing follicle; the activity of these cells decreases, for reasons that are not clear, prior to ovulation. The increasing plasma oestrogen concentration 'triggers' the discharge of the hypothalamic releasing factors and consequently the pituitary with a resultant sudden mid-cycle increase in FSH and LH concentration (*see Figure 7.2*). Approximately 24 hours after the surge in LH release ovulation takes place. In the follicular phase oestradiol also prepares the female genital tract for sperm migration and pregnancy by:

1. Increasing the cervical secretion of mucus.
2. Stimulating uterine endometrial proliferation.
3. Modifying the motility of the fallopian tube to facilitate the entry of an ovum into the ampulla.

After ovulation the granulosa cells of the ruptured follicle undergo a process of hypertrophy and hyperplasia (luteinization); the developing corpus luteum is also invaded by a number of theca interna cells. The corpus luteum secretes both oestradiol and 17-α-hydroxyprogesterone but the principal hormone secreted by the corpus luteum is progesterone, and this reaches a maximum at

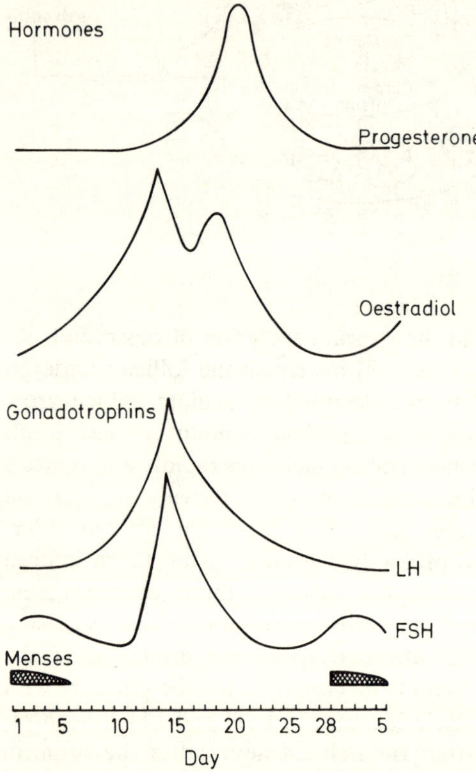

Figure 7.2 Sequential changes in blood gonadotrophins and hormones during the normal menstrual cycle. (For concentration changes of these hormones see the text)

approximately five to seven days after ovulation. Further hormone developments are dependent on the fate of the ovum. If fertilization has not taken place the activity of the corpus luteum begins to decline with a reduction in the plasma concentrations of progesterone, oestradiol and 17-α-hydroxyprogesterone. As the circulating plasma concentrations of these hormones decrease towards the end of the cycle their inhibitory effect on the hypothalamus is diminished with a rise in FSH secretion, and this is followed by the onset of a new cycle. The regression in activity of the corpus luteum is possibly caused by the release of a prostaglandin ($F_{2\alpha}$) from the progesterone – and oestrogen – primed endometrium. The prostaglandin passes directly from the uterine vein into the ovarian cavity without entering the systemic circulation and is not measurable therefore in the blood. If fertilization of the ovum has taken place the resultant blastocyte reaches the uterine cavity at approximately the peak of the post-ovulatory progesterone concentration and it is ready to implant at this stage. Progesterone helps to provide the type of endometrium suitable for implantation. If implantation takes place successfully a new hormone appears, human chorionic gonadotrophin (HCG), which maintains the function of the corpus luteum of pregnancy.

Post-menopausal stage

The menopause is associated with a decline in ovarian activity. The reduction in negative feedback is associated with hyperactivity of the hypothalamus and pituitary with marked increases in plasma LH and FSH concentration which continue throughout the menopause.

Specimens and normal range values

No special patient preparation is required for these assays for which 5 ml of venous blood in a heparin container is required.

FSH and LH (*see* page 17)

Oestradiol-17-β

Oestradiol-17-β is produced by the ovaries and the placenta in females of reproductive age; a small amount of oestrone is produced by the adrenal cortex which is converted in the circulation into oestradiol. As virtually all of the oestrogen produced in females of reproductive age is oestradiol measurement of its plasma concentration provides a valuable index of ovarian functional activity.

Normal range values for plasma are:

Follicular phase	110–370 pmol/ℓ
Peri-ovulatory	370–1470 pmol/ℓ
Luteal phase	180–550 pmol/ℓ
Post-menopausal	20–70 pmol/ℓ

Progesterone

The assay of plasma progesterone provides an index of luteal function. The plasma concentration varies with the stage of the menstrual cycle – the absence of an increase in concentration of this hormone in the luteal phase (peak value approximately day 24) is indicative of either an anovulatory cycle or a defective corpus luteum.

Normal range values for progesterone are:

Follicular phase	0.6–2.9 nmol/ℓ
Luteal phase	9.5–95 nmol/ℓ
Post-menopausal	0.1–1.0 nmol/ℓ

Pregnanediol

Pregnanediol is the main metabolite of progesterone and is excreted in the urine. In the non-pregnant female who is infertile the urinary assay of this compound is of value in the assessment of ovarian function if a plasma progesterone assay is not available. It should be undertaken during the luteal phase. This assay is of no value in the investigation of oligomenorrhoea and amenorrhoea.

Normal range values for pregnanediol are:

Females	
Folicular phase	0–1.6 µmol/24h
Luteal phase	>6 µmol/24h
Post-menopausal	0.4–2.8 µmol/24h
Males	0–3.0 µmol/24h

Urine total oestrogens in the non-pregnant

The assay technique used measures oestriol, oestrone and oestradiol; either of the first two of these may be the predominant urinary oestrogen and both are equally important in the assessment of oestrogen production. A major use of this assay is the monitoring of the therapeutic response to techniques used to induce ovulation.

A complete 24-hour collection of urine is required in a container to which has been added 10 ml of 2% boric acid as a preservative.

A number of drugs cause interference with this assay and they should be stopped if at all possible. The drugs include ACTH, corticosteroids, ampicillin, glucose, mandelamine, meprobromate, senna and stilboestrol which cause false low values, while barbiturates, chlorpromazine and diuretics may cause false high values.

Normal values are:

Females
    Follicular phase   25–105 nmol/24h
    Ovulatory mid-cycle peak140–350 nmol/24h
    Luteal phase   105–350 nmol/24h
Males   25–90 nmol/24h

Urine total oestrogens in pregnancy

The assay or urinary oestriol as total pregnancy oestrogens in maternal urine provides an index of the well-being of the fetal-placental unit. Oestriol is synthesized in the adrenal of the fetus, hydroxylated in its liver and then, after aromatization in the placenta, is excreted in the maternal urine. In the event of either placental or fetal malfunction there is a fall in the levels which normally rise progressively through pregnancy and provide one indication that early delivery may be necessary.

Dynamic tests

Clomiphene stimulation test

Clomiphene citrate is given orally for seven days starting on the third day of the menstrual cycle if menstruating and this constitutes day 1 of the test. A venous blood sample for LH and progesterone assay is collected prior to the start of treatment.

The dose of clomiphene citrate used is normally 2 mg/kg/day to the nearest 50 mg in divided doses. Some workers, however, prefer to do a first test in patients with amenorrhoea with a total oral dose of 50 mg/day for seven days followed by, if necessary, a second test using a total dose of 100 mg/day for the seven days.

On test days 3, 5, 8 and 11 (or 12 if 11 falls on a Sunday) further venous blood samples are collected for LH assay.

On test day 21 a venous blood sample should be collected for progesterone assay.

If the hypothalamic–pituitary– ovarian axis is intact there is a normal response which is indicated by a rise in plasma LH to a value of 6 U/ℓ or more during the test period days 1–11. A failure in ovulatory response is also shown by a lack of a post-ovulatory (day 21) peak in plasma progesterone.

LH–RH test (*see* also page 20)

This test is of value in the endocrine investigation of patients who are suspected of not ovulating or who are not menstruating. An absent or impaired response suggests that there is either a primary or secondary abnormality of the pituitary gonadotrophs. If there is a normal or exaggerated response to LH–RH then further information on the functional state of the axis is provided by a clomiphene stimulation test. Females with a normal LH–RH response may be divided into those with disturbed cyclical gonadotrophin release who respond to clomiphene, and those with a block in releasing hormone production who do not respond to clomiphene. In females with primary ovarian failure the exaggerated response to LH–RH is confirmed by high basal LH values which are unaffected by the administration of clomiphene.

Human menopausal gonadotrophin stimulation

Human menopausal gonadotrophin contains equal amounts of both FSH and LH. It is used in sequence with human chorionic gonadotrophin (HCG) for the treatment of infertility which has been attributed to a failure of ovulation*. The aim of human menopausal gonadotrophin treatment is to induce follicular maturation and endometrial proliferation. A single dose of HCG is then given to 'trigger' ovulation and corpus luteum formation. If an adequate response to human menopausal gonadotrophin is achieved and HCG is given the patient is advised to have coitus both on that day and the subsequent day (days 8 and 9 – in the method detailed below). The dosage of human menopausal gonadotrophin must be adjusted for each individual patient and this can be achieved by measurement of the urine total non-pregnancy oestrogens (or blood).

The indications for human menopausal gonadotrophin stimulation are primary or secondary amenorrhoea and anovulation with either regular or irregular cycles. Although there are no absolute contra-indications, human menopausal gonadotrophin should not be used on patients with the following conditions:

1. Ovarian dysgenesis and premature menopause.
2. Abnormal reproductive organs which are incompatible with fertility even if ovulation is induced.
3. Endocrine disorders that of themselves can cause anovulation.
4. Pituitary tumours (prior to irradiation or surgery) or other intracranial lesions.
5. Organic causes for abnormal bleeding patterns.
6. Infertility in the partner – unless it is treatable.

Method   Three equal dose injections of human menopausal gonadotrophin are given on three alternate days (days 1, 3 and 5) followed by a single injection of 10 000 units of HCG on day 8 if indicated. The latter is dependent on the response as measured by the urinary total non-pregnancy oestrogens in a 24-hour specimen collected on day 6 when compared with a 24-hour collection on the day prior to commencement of injections (day 0) starting dose schedule:

1. Amenorrhoeic patients – 1050 units human menopausal gonadotrophin (5 ampoules of Pergonal) on days 1, 3 and 5

*Human gonadotrophin obtained from either urine or the pituitary may be used. There are proprietary preparations, e.g. Pergonal (G.D. Searle).

2. Menstruating patients – 750 units human menopausal gonadotrophin (3 ampoules of Pergonal) on days 1, 3 and 5.

The dose used in subsequent courses is gauged from the initial response. The responses to human menopausal gonadotrophin as assessed by urine total oestrogens are shown in *Table 7.1*.

Table 7.1 Responses to human menopausal gonadotrophin

Response		Urine total oestrogens Difference day 6–Basal (nmol/24h)
None	rise less than	35
Poor	rise between	38–104
Adequate	rise between	107–434
High	rise between	438–1730
Excessive	rise greater than	1730

An adequate response based on blood oestradiol values is to a value between 1100 to 3000 pmol/ℓ (300 to 800 pg/ml).

Clinical considerations

Although ovarian disorders may be considered under the two major headings of hypofunction and hyperfunction, in clinical practice they are usually considered under the headings of amenorrhoea, infertility, precocious puberty, hirsutism and virilism.

Amenorrhoea

The term 'primary' is used if the patient has never had a period and 'secondary' if menstruation, having previously occurred, has stopped. The only value of these terms is that some patients with either chromosomal abnormalities or malformations of the genital tract fall into the primary category, otherwise the age of onset of symptoms is the more important and the primary/secondary terminology can be discarded.

The causes of amenorrhoea include the following:

1. Pregnancy.
2. Hypothalamic:
   (*a*) Psychological stress

(*b*) Anorexia nervosa

(*c*) Pseudocyesis – either fear or desire of pregnancy

(*d*) Frohlich's syndrome (dystrophia adiposogenitalis) – a hypothalamic disturbance in which there is amenorrhoea, genital hypoplasia and obesity

(*e*) Hyperprolactinaemia

3. Pituitary:

   (*a*) Sheehan's syndrome (post-partum pituitary necrosis)

   (*b*) Pituitary tumours – loss of gonadotrophins with amenorrhoea is often the first clinical evidence of pituitary damage

   (*c*) Trauma

   (*d*) Vascular lesions.

4. Adrenal:

   (*a*) Cushing's syndrome

   (*b*) Adrenogenital syndrome.

5. Ovarian:

   (*a*) Turner's syndrome (ovarian dysgenesis)

   (*b*) Disorders of sex differentiation – male and female pseudo-hermaphroditism

   (*c*) Premature ovarian failure

   (*d*) Ovarian tumours which secrete an excess of androgens

   (*e*) Stein–Leventhal (polycystic ovary) syndrome

6. 'Post-oral-contraceptive pill', amenorrhoea: this is common for a few months after stopping the pill and is presumably the result of prolonged hypothalamic pituitary suppression. In others, menstruation may not return and the cause is uncertain but hyperprolactinaemia probably accounts for one-third of these cases.

7. Drugs:

   (*a*) Antidepressants (tricyclics)

   (*b*) Phenothiazines.

   (*c*) Some antihypertensive agents.

8. Hyperthyroidism

9. Diabetes mellitus

10.Obesity

Plan of investigation

Secondary amenorrhoea

1. FSH (or LH–RH) test.

2. Skull X-ray for pituitary fossa.
3. Serum prolactin.
4. Clomiphene test.

Primary amenorrhoea

1. FSH and LH (or LH–RH) test.
2. Buccal smear or Karyotype.
3. Skull X-ray for pituitary fossa.
4. X-ray for bone age.

Note: Failure to respond to LH–RH indicates disease of pituitary.
Response to LH–RH but not to clomiphene indicates lesion above pituitary–usually hypothalamic.

The endocrinological investigation of amenorrhoea is usually undertaken by the simultaneous basal measurement of those variables which would either confirm or exclude the diagnosis of the various listed causative conditions. The use of either clomiphene or a LH–RH test should *not* be undertaken until a basal FSH assay is available, as a high value is indicative of primary ovarian failure.

Infertility

The disorders that cause infertility are essentially the same as those that cause amenorrhoea and oligomenorrhoea with, in addition, a number of anatomical and pathological abnormalities of the genital tract. It should, however, be remembered that male infertility is responsible for nearly one-third of infertile marriages.

The endocrinological investigation of infertility must include the estimation of LH, FSH, oestradiol and plasma progesterone (preferably on approximately day 24, to confirm ovulation, although the only certain confirmation of ovulation is conception). The patient's thyroid, adrenal and androgen status should also be assessed and plasma prolactin measured.

Hyperprolactinaemic hypogonadism

This constitutes a group of infertile patients who have high prolactin values sometimes in association with galactorrhoea. It is most common in patients with pituitary adenomas, post-partum or post-oral-contraceptive amenorrhoea, polycystic ovaries, and may occasionally occur in patients with either hypothalamic disease or primary hypothyroidism; it may also occasionally be idiopathic. The precise mechanism whereby hyperprolactinaemia leads to hypogonadism is unknown, but prolactin-induced blockade of gonadotrophins at gonadal level is at least partly responsible.

Precocious puberty

The development of secondary sexual characteristics before the age of eight years may be classified as precocious and warrants endocrinological investigation.

The causes include:

1. Hypothalamic or pituitary tumours, and tumours in the region of the pineal, cause precocious puberty by hypothalamic pressure.
2. Ovarian tumours secreting an excess of oestrogens cause a precocious pseudo puberty. These include tumours of the granulosa and theca cells, luteomas and the highly malignant teratomas and chorionepitheliomas. All of these tumours produce oestrogen, and in the case of the last three progesterone is also secreted.
3. Adrenal tumours only rarely produce oestrogens (more usually androgens).
4. Polyostotic fibrous dysplasia. A syndrome characterized by precocious puberty, characteristic cystic bone lesions on radiology, patches of skin pigmentation and occasionally hyperthyroidism. The skin pigmentation and bone lesions are usually unilateral.
5. Post-infections, for example, meningitis, toxoplasmosis.
6. Hormone-secreting non-endocrine tumours – hepatomas and hepatoblastomas.

The endocrinological investigation of precocious puberty should include not only estimation of the oestrogens and gonadotrophins (FSH and LH) but also thyroid hormones.

Hirsuties and virilism

Hirsuties may be defined as an excessive growth of hair which may occur on the face, body or limbs. The excessive hair growth may present without other abnormalities, or it may be accompanied by other features of virilization such as clitoral hypertrophy, thinning of the scalp hair with temporal recession and oligomenorrhoea or amenorrhoea. The underlying disorder in hirsuties may be, although not necessarily, due to a disorder of androgen metabolism, whereas virilism is indicative of an excessive production of androgens. The ovary normally produces a very small amount of androgens. In some disease states there is an excessive production of testosterone while in others androstenedione. The latter is in the normal metabolic pathway of both oestrone and testosterone; although it has a lesser masculinizing activity than testosterone it can be converted into this hormone in the liver and at other sites in the body. There may also be an increased secretion of dehydroepiandosterone (DHA) – a weak androgen – or its sulphate conjugate (DHA–S).

The causes of hirsutism include:

1. Constitutional or 'physiological':
   (*a*) racial, familial or idiopathic
   (*b*) post-menopausal
2. Drug-induced: corticosteroids, androgens, anabolic hormones, progestogens, phenytoin, minoxidil and diazoxide.
3. Andrenocortical:
   (*a*) Congenital adrenal hyperplasia
   (*b*) Adrenocortical tumours
   In some tumours of the adrenal cortex, particularly carcinomas but also with some adenomas, there may be virilism without cushingoid features – excessive production of DHA, androsterone and also testosterone.
4. Ovarian:
   (*a*) Polycystic ovary syndrome – the most common ovarian cause – usually associated with infertility and menstrual irregularities
   (*b*) Androgen-secreting tumours – arrhenoblastomas and hilus cell tumours, both of which are rare
   (*c*) Maldevelopment – ovarian dysgenesis

The causes of virilism are identical with the exception of constitutional or 'physiological'.

The endocrinological investigation of hirsutism and virilism should include plasma testosterone and the urine excretion of 17-oxosteroids together with other investigations which would be appropriate for the diagnosis of the causative conditions listed, and which may be indicated by the history and clinical examination.

Of debatable value in the differential diagnosis of patients with hirsutism and virilism is the dexamethasone suppression test (*see* page 38) in a modified manner with collection of urine for 17-oxosteroids and blood for testosterone assay. The test schedule is modified as shown in *Table 7.2*.

Table 7.2

Day	Dose	24h Urine 17-oxo-steroids	Plasma testo-sterone
1	Basal	+	+
2	Basal	+	
3	Dexamethasone 0.5 mg q.i.d.	+	
4	Dexamethasone 0.5 mg q.i.d.	+	
5	Dexamethasone 0.5 mg q.i.d.	+	+
6	—		+

+ Blood and urine collections (blood collections at 0900 hours)

In a normal response the urine 17-oxosteroids and plasma testosterone will fall by more than 50% of their basal values – and this will often occur in patients with idiopathic hirsuties, polycystic ovaries and congenital adrenal hyperplasia. Theoretically, if the source of androgen is adrenal it should be suppressed by dexamethasone. This constantly occurs with congenital adrenal hyperplasia but not with tumours of the adrenal cortex. Furthermore, suppression of ovarian production of androgens not infrequently occurs in the polycystic ovary syndrome and in idiopathic hirsutism. Conversely, a rise in urinary androgens after HCG would, theoretically, indicate an ovarian source but adrenal androgens are often increased following HCG. The dexamethasone suppression test is therefore not a reliable indicator of the source of androgen production.

8 Testicular disorders

Physiology

The testis of reproductive man serves two functions–spermatogenesis, and the formation and secretion of androgens. The latter are essential for spermatogenesis and for the functioning of the secretory epithelium; hormone production is independent of sperm production.

Testicular function is under the control of the pituitary gonadotrophins LH and FSH, although in the male LH should be more appropriately called *interstitial-cell-stimulating hormone (ICSH)*. There is some evidence to suggest that both LH and FSH act on the testis to initiate spermatogenesis and that only LH is required for continuation once it has commenced. In the male, FSH is, however, usually regarded as being the prime regulator of spermatogenesis, with LH acting indirectly through the action of testosterone. The release of the pituitary gonadotrophins is controlled by the hypothalamic gonadotrophin-releasing hormone (LH/FSH–RH); testosterone exerts a negative feedback control on LH secretion (*see* page 17), the regulation of FSH secretion is controversial and possibly involves an inhibitory factor from the seminiferous tubules (inhibin).

Spermatogenesis is a complex process which takes place in the seminiferous tubules and has three principal phases:

1. Spermatocyte formation–the stem cells or spermatogonia undergo mitotic division and produce the primary spermatocytes.

2. Spermatid formation – primary spermatocytes then undergo a meiotic division to produce secondary spermatocytes, at this stage the chromosome number is reduced from the diploid (46) to the haploid (23) number and the X and Y chromosomes are secregated. The secondary spermatocytes then undergo a second meiotic division and spermatids (haploid) are produced.
3. Spermiogenesis – cytological changes take place in the spermatids and sperm is formed. Sperm are released from the epithelium into the lumina of the seminiferous tubules and are then, by peristaltic action, transported into the epididymal ducts which serve as sperm reservoirs (the transit time is from 14 to 20 days). Sperm are non-motile until they reach the ducts, by which time they have matured.

Testosterone is produced in the interstitial or Leydig cells and is the most potent of the three principal testicular hormones; the other two being *androstenedione* and *dehydroepiandrosterone* (DHEA). Testosterone appears to require conversion to *5-α-dihydrotestosterone (DHT)* which is a much more biologically active form; the conversion occurs both in the circulation and in the peripheral target tissues. Testosterone and DHT are transported in the blood bound loosely to carrier proteins, mainly a globulin – sex-hormone-binding globulin (SHBG). Androgenic activity is considered to be a function of the free plasma androgen concentration. The testis is also the major source of oestrogen in males. A small amount of oestradiol or oestrone is produced by the testis as such but most of the testicular oestrogen is the result of the conversion of testosterone to oestradiol. A small amount of oestrogen is of adrenal origin. The physiological effects of testosterone can be divided into androgenic and anabolic although both are really anabolic.

The classical androgenic functions as such are:

1. Normal differentiation of the external genitalia in the fetus.
2. Normal spermatogenesis.
3. Development at puberty and subsequent maintenance of secondary sexual characteristics.

The anabolic effects are:

1. Increase in muscle mass, strength and tone.
2. Stimulation of bone growth with, at a later date, epiphyseal closure.
3. A stimulatory role in erythrocyte production and a permissive role in the formation and secretion of erythropoietin.

Testosterone is metabolized in the liver with the other androgens to androsterone, epiandrosterone and etiochlanolone. These compounds are excreted in the urine in conjugation with glucuronic and sulphuric acid and together with DHEA and DHEA sulphate are the principal compounds that constitute the urinary 17-oxosteroids. Approximately two-thirds of the urine 17-oxosteroids, however, come from the adrenal gland and only one-half of the remainder is a metabolite of testosterone. The importance of these various metabolite contributions to the urine 17-oxosteroids is that major changes can occur in testicular testosterone secretion without a marked change in urine 17-oxosteroid excretion.

Specimens and normal range values

Plasma LH and FSH (*see* page 17)

Plasma testosterone

A 10 ml venous blood sample should be collected into a heparin tube. The specimen should be taken to the laboratory immediately after collection for separation. The patient need not be fasting, but there is evidence of both a physiological variation in concentration through the day as well as the occurrence of episodic 'bursts' of hormone secretion. The concentration measured in plasma is dependent not only on production rate but also on the concentration of sex-hormone-binding globuilin. Increased concentrations of the binding protein may be found after treatment with oestrogens, in pregnancy and in females taking oral contraceptives:

Males   10.4–34.6 nmol/ℓ
Females   0.7–2.8 nmol/ℓ

Urine 17-oxosteroids (*see* page 31)

Dynamic tests

Clomiphene stimulation test

Clomiphene is thought to act essentially through competition at the hypothalamic receptor centres, stimulating the release of LH/FSH–RH and gonadotrophins by negative feedback. The normal response to clomiphene is therefore dependent on a functionally intact hypothalamic–pituitary–gonadal axis.

Method (males)   Day 1: collect venous blood sample for FSH and LH. Start oral clomiphene citrate in a daily dosage of 2 mg/kg body weight (to the nearest 50 mg) in a divided twice daily dose; this is continued for a total of seven days.
Days 3, 5 and 8: collect venous blood samples for FSH and LH.

Normal response   The normal response is an increment to above the normal range in FSH and LH values.

Side-effects   The patient may experience visual phenomena – either peripheral field 'flickering' or central haloes – and occasionally some become depressed, if the side-effects are severe the test should be stopped. The test is contraindicated in patients with a history of a recent depressive illness or liver disease.

HCG stimulation test

Human chorionic gonadotrophin (HCG) stimulates interstitial cells and can be used as a test of their ability to secrete testosterone.

Method   Day 1: collect venous blood sample for testosterone at 0900 hours. Inject intramuscularly a dose of 1500 units of HCG.
Day 2, 3 and 4: repeat the intramuscular injection of 1500 units of HCG.

Day 4: collect venous blood sample for testosterone at 0900 hours prior to the HCG injection.
Day 5: collect further blood for testosterone.

Normal response   This is an increase in plasma testosterone to above the upper limit of the normal range in at least one of the test samples.

In primary testicular disease there is either a reduced or absent response.

In hypogonadotrophism a normal response may be obtained.

Diagnostic considerations

Disturbance of testicular function may be considered clinically under three headings – infertility, hypogonadism and precocious puberty.

Infertility

Infertility is usually due to disturbances in semen production, impotence, abnormalities in the partner, poor sexual technique and only rarely to androgen deficiency. If there is a severe degree of damage to the seminiferous tubules the FSH concentration in increased. The FSH and LH concentrations will, however, be reduced if there is a failure of gonadotrophin formation or release in patients with either hypothalamic or pituitary disorders.

Plasma testosterone concentration is normal in patients with primary disorders of the seminiferous tubules and decreased in patients with hypothalamic–pituitary disorders. The assay of FSH, LH and testosterone should be estimated both under basal conditions and, if necessary, after stimulation with clomiphene or HCG. The full investigation of male infertility is outside the scope of this book but must include not only endocrine assessment but also semen analysis, karyotype, possibly testicular biopsy, as well as a full clinical history, examination and investigation of the patient, and the female partner.

Hypogonadism

The clinical features of testicular disease with androgen deficiency, due to failure of the interstitial cells, depends on the age of the patient. In the child, the presentation is either a delay in the onset of puberty or the development of eunuchoidal features. In an adult the presentation is initially that of a reduction in libido and potency followed after a variable time by regression of secondary sexual characteristics.

The diagnostic biochemical findings are a low plasma testosterone with a failure of response in an HCG stimulation test. Maturation of the hypothalamic–pituitary–gonadal axis often occurs before the onset of puberty and the LH–RH test (*see* page 20) can be used to assess the degree of maturation of this axis in patients with delayed puberty. This test is also of value in the differential diagnosis of primary gonadal failure from hypothalamic–pituitary disease in these patients. In the adult patient with primary gonadal failure the basal values of FSH and LH are usually increased with an enhanced response in an LH–RH test.

Precocious puberty (*see* also page 77)

This term includes both true precocious puberty, in which there is an early maturation of the normal hypothalamic–pituitary–gonadal axis; and pseudo-precocious puberty, in which there is development of secondary sexual characteristics in the absence of gonadal maturation. The latter condition is due to the overproduction of either oestrogens or androgens from the gonads, adrenals or from tumours which contain gonadal tissue (teratomas).

The clinical features of precocious puberty may appear early in life with, in males, penile growth, development of pubic hair, rapid muscular and skeletal development and premature fusion of epiphyses leading ultimately to a reduction in height. In the pseudo state normal testicular development does not take place and spermatogenesis is absent.

The biochemical features include an increase in urinary 17-oxosteroid excretion, with increased plasma LH and FSH when compared with children of comparable age. In pseudo-precocious puberty the pituitary gonadotrophins are either normal or decreased while plasma testosterone is increased.

9 Disorders of calcium homeostasis

Physiology

The normal steady-state regulation of calcium includes diet, physiochemical mechanisms and hormones; the latter are dominant. Disturbances, as a consequence of disease states, in any of these three control systems are associated with disorders of calcium homeostasis. The latter are usually manifested as either hypercalcaemia or hypocalcaemia.

The ultimate source of the body's calcium and phosphorus is the diet. Dietary intake and the digestive mechanisms control the amounts of these two ions that are available for intestinal absorption. In the child calcium and phosphorus are retained for skeletal growth, in the adult only enough is retained to offset obligatory losses, normally in urine and faeces. During pregnancy and lactation extra losses occur by transfer to the fetus for the formation of the skeleton and for milk production. In the kidney excretion is controlled by renal tubular reabsorption and in the bowel, to a lesser extent, by endogenous secretion. Both the child and the adult need, therefore, to adapt calcium and phosphorus absorption and balance to the requirements of the skeleton in the face of variations in dietary intake and excretion. The adaptive mechanisms involve variations in hormone secretion rates. In addition to the requirements for the maintenance of the skeleton, there is the over-riding need to maintain a constant concentration of ionized calcium which is essential for normal neuromuscular function and probably for other cell functions such as secretion and transport. A constant concentration of plasma phosphorus may also be needed.

The physiochemical factors include those that may potentially affect the rate of ion exchange, between the bone crystal surface and the extracellular fluid compartment, and those that are involved in skeletal homeostasis. The latter include weight bearing and muscle activity. Most of the body's calcium (99%) and much of its phosphorus (85%) are present in bone; anything that affects the rate of either bone deposition or resorption can cause a disturbance in steady-state calcium regulation.

The hormones that are essential in the steady-state regulation of calcium and phosphorus are parathyroid hormone (PTH), 1,25-dihydroxycholecalciferol (1,25-DHCC) and calcitonin. The precise physiological role of the latter, in man, requires further clarification. A number of other hormones are also involved in overall calcium and skeletal homeostasis and these include: growth hormone, prolactin, the sex steroids, thyroxine and cortisol. All of these hormones have only subsidiary roles. The essential hormones exert their control of calcium homeostasis by their actions on:

1. The rate of calcium deposition or mobilization from bone
2. The urinary excretion of calcium
3. The rate of absorption of calcium from the intestinal tract.

A fall in the concentration of ionized calcium, in plasma, is the major stimulus to PTH production and secretion. A negative feedback mechanism between plasma calcium and PTH secretion is responsible for the relative constancy of plasma calcium concentration. The calcium-sensitive receptors in the parathyroid gland also respond to changes in the plasma ionized magnesium concentration. Although a fall in plasma magnesium concentration can stimulate PTH, paradoxically at low levels of plasma magnesium PTH production is reduced since magnesium ion is essential for secretion. The parathyroid cell responds immediately to changes in plasma calcium by increasing production and secretion. Both the maximal output and the basal secretion rate are proportional to the glandular mass. Within the parathyroid gland the initial biosynthetic product is a single chain polypeptide of 115 amino acids–*Pre-proparathyroid Hormone*. The latter is immediately converted to the storage form–*Proparathyroid Hormone*. Prior to release from the gland the latter is converted into *Parathyroid Hormone* – a single polypeptide chain, consisting of 84 amino acids, which has a molecular weight of 9500 daltons; this may also be termed *intact-PTH*. The major portion of PTH in the circulation appears to consist of one or more smaller peptide fragments of intact-PTH with longer half-lives than the intact hormone. An understanding of the steps in the biosynthesis and degradation of PTH is essential for the interpretation of hormone concentration in disease states, particularly in patients with chronic renal failure.

The biological actions of PTH involve target tissues in the kidney, bone and gastrointestinal tract. At the target tissues PTH acts on specific cell membrane receptors, linked to adenyl cyclase; this releases cyclic adenosine monophosphate intracellularly which transmits the stimulus within the cell. The action of PTH on the kidney is accompanied by an increased excretion of urinary cyclic adenosine monophosphate (cyclic AMP); this effect is of differential diagnostic value.

The biological actions of PTH on the kidney involve the handling of calcium, phosphate and other ions together with an effect on the production of 1,25-DHCC. In the absence of PTH, 97% of the filtered load of calcium is reabsorbed by the renal tubules. PTH increases the tubular reabsorption of calcium, raises the renal calcium threshold and hence the plasma calcium concentration. In the absence of PTH over 90% of the filtered phosphate is reabsorbed. PTH decreases the tubular reabsorption of phosphate, lowers the renal threshold and allows the same excretion of phosphate at a lower plasma concentration; the overall effect is to cause a reduction in plasma phosphorus concentration. It also affects the renal tubular handling of hydrogen ions and causes a decrease in the tubular reabsorption of bicarbonate with a consequent alkaline urine. PTH increases the renal tubular reabsorption of sodium and magnesium, and also has an affect on cholecalciferol metabolism which stimulates the renal production of 1,25-DHCC from its precursor 25-hydroxycholecalciferol (25-HCC). The biological action of PTH causes an increase in bone resorption; both the mineral and collagen components are broken down and released into the circulation. Since proline in collagen is not re-utilized, the urinary excretion rate of hydroxyproline can be used as an index of the action of PTH on bone. Increased bone mineralization, associated with increased resorption, is reflected on histological examination by excessive calcifying osteoid and in plasma by an increase in bone alkaline phosphatase activity.

Cholecalciferol is formed in the skin photochemically from 7-dehydrocholesterol. The first step in the conversion of cholecalciferol, to its ultimate biologically active form, occurs in the liver with hydroxylation at the C-25 position and the formation of 25-hydroxycholecalciferol (25-HCC). The latter is further hydroxylated in the kidney at the C-1 position with the formation of 1,25-dihydroxycholecalciferol (1,25-DHCC) which is the major biologically active metabolite or hormonal form of cholecalciferol. The kidney is the production site of another dihydroxymetabolite, 24,25-dihydroxycholecalciferol (24,25-DHCC). Although the latter metabolite may have a role in calcium and phosphate metabolism this role remains to be defined, as does the role of other dihydroxy and trihydroxy metabolites. In hypocalcaemic situations renal synthesis is orientated to 1-hydroxylation and 1,25-DHCC production with a transition to 24,25-DHCC production as the plasma calcium concentration increases up into the normal range. The production of 1,25-DHCC is controlled by two systems:

1. Plasma calcium, phosphate, PTH and 1,25-DHCC itself; this system regulates 1,25-DHCC production to suit the short-term needs for calcium and phosphorus and is under negative feedback control.
2. This is probably designed for longer term homeostasis and consists of growth hormone, prolactin and the sex steroids, but which of these stimuli have the major control in any particular situation is as yet ill-defined.

The major biological sites of action of 1,25-DHCC are bone, and the gastrointestinal tract where it acts on specific nuclear cellular receptors. The active transport of calcium and phosphorus across the gut wall is virtually zero in the absence of 1,25-DHCC, although calcium and phosphorus can still passively diffuse across if the dietary intake is high enough. The active transport of calcium and of phosphorus across the gut wall is increased by 1,25-DHCC and causes an increase in their plasma concentrations.

The uncalcified osteoid, which is present in patients with rickets and osteomalacia, is remineralized following treatment with 1,25-DHCC. Mineralization may involve extracellular calcium and phosphate concentrations and the factors that regulate the coupling process between resorption and mineralization. The increase in bone resorption is clearly seen following over-treatment with either vitamin D or its biologically active metabolites. Hypercalcaemia in this situation is caused not only by increased intestinal calcium absorption but also by increased bone resorption. Other tissues on which 1,25-DHCC has a biological action include the parathyroid glands, kidneys and muscle. Specific receptors for vitamin D are present in the cells of the parathyroid glands and parathyroid secretion rate can be altered by vitamin D metabolites in experimental animals. When 1,25-DHCC is given therapeutically to hypoparathyroid patients there is an eventual increase in renal tubular reabsorption of calcium and decrease in tubular reabsorption of phosphate with consequent respective changes in their plasma concentrations. Proximal muscle weakness is a striking feature of vitamin D deficiency and is relieved on treatment with 1,25-DHCC.

Specimens and normal range values

For the assay of total plasma calcium, magnesium, phosphorus, total protein and albumin concentrations, and alkaline phosphatase activity 5 ml samples of venous blood should be sent to the laboratory in sterile containers.

Calcium (total)

Ideally the patient should be fasting prior to collection of blood for calcium estimations, but this is not essential as increments in serum calcium concentration of the order of only, at the most, 0.13–0.20 mmol/ℓ occur during a normal working day, after either the intake of normal meals or large oral calcium loads. The use of a protein correction factor, specifically for albumin concentration, is of value. The use of such a factor is of importance in comparing the calcium values in any one patient over a period of time when alterations in total serum protein and albumin concentration may occur. An approximate calcium correction factor for variations in albumin concentration is the addition or subtraction of 0.025 mmol/ℓ of calcium to the measured total calcium for each 1.0 g/ℓ of albumin below or above, respectively, a value of 40 g/ℓ.

Normal range values for total serum calcium concentration are 2.10–2.60 mmol/ℓ.

Calcium (ionized)

The ionized calcium fraction is considered to be the physiologically active portion which is both the controlled and controlling mechanism in the secretion of PTH and 1,25-DHCC. The diagnostic value of the measurement of ionized calcium concentration as a routine procedure in patients with disorders of calcium homeostasis is controversial. The latter view is based on the observation that in the majority of patients the ionized calcium has a constant percentage relationship to the total concentration. The main indications for ionized calcium measurement are in the assessment of calcium status in patients with:

1. Altered albumin concentrations.
2. Multiple myelomatosis.
3. With recurrent renal stones and normal total serum calcium who may have primary hyperparathyroidism.
4. During open heart surgery with hypothermia.

For the assay of ionized calcium concentration a minimum of 3 ml of venous blood should be collected anaerobically into a heparinized syringe. The latter should be placed on ice and taken immediately to the laboratory.

Normal range values are blood ionized calcium concentration 1.05–1.25 mmol/ℓ.

Plasma phosphorus

Because of action of parathyroid hormone in blocking the net tubular reabsorption of phosphate, hypophosphataemia has been considered, in the past, to be an important distinguishing feature of patients with hypercalcaemia due to primary hyperparathyroidism when compared with patients with hypercalcaemia due to other causes. In primary hyperparathyroidism, however, consistently low values for plasma phosphorus concentration are usually the exception rather than the rule, even in the presence of normal renal function. A consistently low plasma phosphorus concentration is highly suggestive of primary hyperparathyroidism, but the diagnosis is *not excluded* in the presence of a normal or high concentration. The changes that occur in the plasma phosphorus concentration in disease states associated with hypocalcaemia are variable.

Normal range values of plasma phosphorus (inorganic) concentration are 1.0–1.5 mmol/ℓ.

Phosphate excretion tests

Several phosphate excretion tests have been reported. These tests are all based on the action of parathyroid hormone at the renal tubular level in blocking net phosphate reabsorption. They were devised prior to the availability of parathyroid hormone assays in an attempt to improve both the diagnostic accuracy in patients with borderline primary hyperparathyroidism and to differentiate patients with hypercalcaemia due to primary hyperparathyroidism from patients with hypercalcaemia due to other causes. The tests have been expressed in a variety of clearance equations and can be divided into groups that involve either simple procedures such as the tubular reabsorption of phosphate (TRP) and the phosphate excretion index (PEI) or more complex procedures such as the theoretical renal phosphate treshold (RPThr) and the maximum tubular reabsorption of phosphate (TmP). If the patients are on a metabolic unit with a controlled phosphate intake, have normal or nearly normal renal function and they do not have glycosuria, these tests may be useful in the diagnosis of borderline cases of primary hyperparathyroidism. Abnormalities in the renal handling of phosphate do, however, also occur in a variety of other conditons which may themselves cause hypercalcaemia. Because of the technical difficulties in performing these tests, some of which require constant infusion, and the need for a rigidly controlled dietary phosphate intake, these tests are of limited differential diagnostic value.

Magnesium

In view of the inter-relationships between the mechanisms involved in the regulation of calcium and magnesium homeostasis the estimation of serum concentration is of value in the assessment of hypocalcaemic states.

Normal range values for serum magnesium concentration are 0.8–1.3 mmol/ℓ.

Serum proteins and albumin

In patients with either hypercalcaemia or hypocalcaemia the routine estimation of total serum protein and albumin concentrations, simultaneously with total calcium, is of diagnostic value in the interpretation of the calcium concentration. Serum protein electrophoresis is of value in the differential diagnosis of hypercalcaemia for the identification of those patients with either sarcoidosis or myelomatosis.

Normal range values for total serum protein and albumin concentration are 60–84 g/ℓ and 35–50 g/ℓ respectively.

Alkaline phosphatase

In the differential diagnosis of hypercalcaemia the estimation of serum alkaline phosphatase activity is of little value in itself. In patients with primary hyperparathyroidism the plasma alkaline phosphatase is correlated with the specific radiological findings of hyperparathyroidism (osteitis fibrosa). In hypocalcaemic patients, in the absence of hepatobiliary disease, an increase in alkaline phosphatase is indicative of osteomalacia or rickets. In the interpretation of alkaline phosphatase values, as a screening test for metabolic bone disease, it is important that the age and sex of the patient is taken into consideration.

Normal range values for serum alkaline phosphatase activity in adults are 20–95 U/ℓ. In children the activity is dependent on age with the highest values (up to 360 U/ℓ) in the first two years of life.

Parathyroid hormone

The phenomenon of immunoheterogenity of circulating PTH is probably the major determinant of the results of serum immunoreactive-PTH (i-PTH) measurement with a given radio-immunoassay procedure. Knowledge of the immunospecificity of the assay being used in i-PTH is crucial to the interpretation of test results as well as the simultaneous serum calcium concentration. The routine assay of i-PTH in an individual blood sample using a procedure that employs an antisera with specificity for the carboxy-terminal region of PTH is of value in the diagnosis of primary hyperparathyroidism and the differential diagnosis of hypercalcaemia. Parathyroid hormone secretion is normally suppressed in hypercalcaemic states, other than primary hyperparathyroidism, so that even a marginal increase in serum i-PTH in association with an increased calcium concentration is suggestive of primary hyperparathyroidism.

Assays that employ antisera with specificity for the amino-terminal region of PTH should be used for multiple venous sampling; these assays reflect acute changes in the secretion rate of PTH. Attempts to localize parathyroid adenomas by selective neck vein catheterization and i-PTH assay on multiple samples should be reserved for those patients who have undergone previous neck surgery and have either persistent or recurrent hypercalcaemia.

For i-PTH assay 5 ml of venous blood should be collected into a sterile container, the latter placed on ice and sent to the laboratory immediately.

Normal range values for i-PTH (carboxy-terminal) are 0.3–1.3 ng/ml with simultaneous serum calcium concentrations of 2.10–2.60 mmol/ℓ and for i-PTH (amino-terminal) 18–40 pg/ml.

25-Hydroxyvitamin D and 1,25-dihydroxycholecalciferol

The assays of 25-hydroxyvitamin D (25-OHD) and 1.25-dihydroxycholecalciferol (1,25-DHCC) are of value in the differential diagnosis of hypercalcaemic and hypocalcaemic states that are either known or considered to be caused by disorders in vitamin D metabolism, e.g., vitamin D overdose; bone disease in chronic renal failure, biliary tract or liver disorders; diphenylhydantoin therapy; etc. The assays of these metabolites are also of value as indices of compliance in the monitoring of therapy with vitamin D metabolites. Serum 1,25-DHCC may be elevated in patients with primary hyperparathyroidism.

For the assay of serum 25-OHD 5 ml of blood in a sterile container should be sent to the laboratory, the container should be wrapped in material that blocks exposure to light. The assay for 25-OHD estimates both $25\text{-}OHD_2$ and $25\text{-}OHD_3$.

Normal range values in adults for 25-hydroxyvitamin D are from 25–95 nmol/ℓ with a lower upper limit during the winter months, and slightly lower values in females when compared with males. In countries where milk is fortified with vitamin D the seasonal variation in 25-OHD does not occur.

Normal range values in adults for 1,25-DHCC are 130–240 pmol/ℓ.

Calcitonin

An increase in serum immunoreactive calcitonin can occur in many disease states, particularly in patients with cancer. Calcitonin assays are useful in the detection of medullary thyroid carcinoma, and in the diagnosis of suspected familial disease (multiple endocrine neoplasia, Type 2). In situations other than medullary thyroid carcinoma there is no evidence that the assay of calcitonin is of diagnostic value.

Urine calcium

The total 24-hour urine calcium excretion rate should be estimated in all patients with hypercalcaemia to confirm the blood findings and also to exclude those very rare patients with hypocalciuric hypercalcaemia. In the majority of hypocalcaemic states urine calcium excretion will be reduced as a consequence of the reduction in the renal filtered load. The estimation of urine calcium excretion is, therefore, of little value in the differential diagnosis of hypocalcaemia. In patients with the Fanconi syndrome urine calcium excretion is increased.

For the measurement of urine calcium excretion an accurately timed urine specimen should be collected (preferably over 24 hours) into a clean container to which hydrochloric acid has been added.

Normal range values for 24-hour urine calcium excretion in an adult are 25–75 mmol/24 hours. The upper limit of the reference range is, however, not clear cut and some normal adults may have values above the upper limit quoted.

Urine hydroxyproline

Hydroxyproline is a non-essential amino acid that occurs almost exclusively in collagen, where it accounts for some 14% of the total amino acids. In patients with primary hyperparathyroidism, or following the administration of parathyroid extract to normal human subjects, the urine excretion of hydroxyproline is increased. This can be attributed to the accelerated bone turnover and collagen degradation. In patients with primary hyperparathyroidism the increase in urine hydroxyproline excretion appears to be a more sensitive index of bone involvement than the plasma alkaline phosphatase activity. As urine hydroxyproline excretion is itself directly correlated with the rate of bone destruction its estimation is of *no value* in the differential diagnosis of patients with hypercalcaemia where bone destruction due to a variety of causes may account for the hypercalcaemia.

Urine cyclic AMP

Urine cyclic AMP (cAMP) excretion represents the target tissue (renal tubule) response to the action of PTH and has been reported to be slightly superior to the i-PTH assay in the differential diagnosis of hypercalcaemia. Relatively poor correlations of urine total cAMP excretion with i-PTH concentration have been reported because of renal impairment. This can be overcome by reporting the results as nephrogenous cAMP which takes into account the glomerular filtration rate and plasma cAMP concentration. In view of the difficulties in measuring the latter an alternative approach is to express the total urine cAMP excretion as a function of the glomerular filtration rate and this may be termed 'nephrogenous' cAMP in comparison to true nephrogenous cAMP.

For the assay of 'nephrogenous' cAMP, a 24-hour or accurately timed urine collection should be sent to the laboratory together with 3 ml of blood in a sterile container for serum creatine estimation.

Normal range values for 'nephrogenous' cAMP are 1.2–3.6 nmol/dl glomerular filtrate.

Dynamic tests

Cortisone suppression test

Following the administration of cortisone there is usually a significant reduction in the hypercalcaemia associated with sarcoidosis, myelomatosis, thyrotoxicosis, vitamin D intoxication and malignant disease which does not occur in the hypercalcaemia associated with primary hyperparathyroidism. Since the original description of this test there have been many reports of patients with proven primary hyperparathyroidism who have shown suppression of their hypercalcaemia, and there also have been reports of patients with hypercalcaemia due to various other causes who have failed to show suppression. In the majority of these conflicting reports the workers have not used the method as originally described and have used other various steroid substitutes. Even when correctly performed, it is recognized that this test is not completely reliable as both suppression of the hypercalcaemia of primary hyperparathyroidism and non-suppression of that due to other causes may occur. Despite this limitation the test is of value in the differential diagnosis of hypercalcaemia when other tests have failed to show definitive patterns. The test as originally described involves the oral administration of a standard 10-day load of cortisone given orally in a dose of 50 mg three times a day; recently hydrocortisone (40 mg three times a day) has been used instead with comparable results to those using cortisone.

Hypercalcaemia

Diagnostic considerations

The symptoms due to hypercalcaemia are vague, non-specific and the same irrespective of the causative mechanism. The symptoms and signs are, in general, proportional to the degree of elevation in the serum calcium concentration and offer no clue to the aetiological mechanism. In any patient with hypercalcaemia there is a risk, if it is allowed to continue, of irreversible renal damage. There is also the risk in hypercalcaemia due to any cause that if there is a marked increase in the serum calcium concentration there may be progression to a hypercalcaemic crisis which has a high mortality unless treated as a medical emergency.

The accurate differential diagnosis of hypercalcaemia is important if rational treatment is to be instituted for the underlying disorder. In many situations a diagnosis can either be made or excluded by either the clinical history or the physical examination. In many patients the differential diagnosis of hypercalcaemia is based on evaluation of their biochemical criteria. The differentiation of the biochemical findings must be related to the mechanisms that cause the increases in plasma calcium concentration.

Carcinoma

The commonest cause of hypercalcaemia is carcinoma. In patients with carcinoma a variety of mechanisms may cause bone dissolution. The most common cause of bone dissolution and consequent hypercalcaemia in patients with carcinoma is the presence of osteolytic bone metastases. In these patients there is an increase in both the serum calcium and phosphorus concentrations.

It has also been established that hypercalcaemia may occur in patients with carcinoma in whom there are no demonstrable metastatic bone lesions, either on radiological bone survey during life or on careful histological examination of the bones at autopsy. In this group of patients other mechanisms have been proposed to account for the hypercalcaemia. These include the secretion of parathyroid hormone-like polypeptides, prostaglandins, osteoclast activating factor and osteolytic sterols.

The secretion by a primary tumour of a polypeptide that has actions similar to those of a naturally occurring hormone is an example of a non-endocrine hormone-secreting tumour. In patients with carcinoma there is evidence that some primary tumours may synthesize a parathyroid hormone-like polypeptide which causes hypercalcaemia and hypophosphataemia; this syndrome has been termed *pseudohyperparathyroidism*.

Pseudohyperparathyroidism is the commonest of the endocrine syndromes associated with bronchial carcinoma and occurs most frequently with tumours of squamous cell origin. The i-PTH like material secreted by these non-endocrine tumours is immunologically different from the hormone present in the serum of patients with primary hyperparathyroidism but it may cross react in some assay systems. The differentiation of patients with pseudohyperparathyroidism from those with primary hyperparathyroidism is of considerable importance, as in the former group there may be a small, relatively symptomless primary neoplasm.

Primary hyperparathyroidism

Primary hyperparathyroidism is a common cause of hypercalcaemia; its accurate diagnosis is important as it is a condition which is amenable to surgical treatment.

In recent years the incidence has increased with the advent of health screening programmes and the discovery of an asymptomatic hypercalcaemia. The reported incidence of subsequently proven primary hyperparathyroidism in these programmes has varied from 1–4/1000 individuals screened. The incidence of primary hyperparathyroidism is higher in women than in men, with a peak between 40 and 70 years of age in both groups.

The laboratory diagnosis of primary hyperparathyroidism is based on the finding of hypercalcaemia with hypophosphataemia, if the latter is present then diagnosis is highly probable, especially with increased or inappropriate values for i-PTH and increased 'nephrogenous' cAMP. In patients with primary hyperparathyroidism there is a tendency to a metabolic acidosis in contrast to a metabolic alkalosis which occurs in patients with hypercalcaemia due to all other causes including those with pseudohyperparathyroidism.

Tertiary hyperparathyroidism may be defined as hypercalcaemia which has developed in a patient with long-standing hypocalcaemia due either to chronic gastrointestinal or renal disease. In the latter group of patients the i-PTH values are 'dramatically' increased and much higher than in primary hyperparathyroidism. The extremely high values for i-PTH in chronic renal failure are accounted for, in part, by a failure of the functionally impaired kidneys to clear biologically inactive peptide fragments from the circulation.

Thiazide diuretics

Although usually mild, hypercalcaemia has been reported to occur in a large proportion of patients receiving diuretics of the thiadizine group. The mechanism of action involves inhibition of the renal tubular reabsorption of sodium; the latter is linked with calcium in an exchange mechanism.

Myelomatosis/leukaemia

In myeloma, hypercalcaemia is common with an incidence of up to 50% of patients. In patients with myelomatosis the hypercalcaemia is in excess of that which can be accounted for either by changes in serum proteins or by the extent of their bone lesions.

Vitamin D intoxication

Vitamin D is a cumulative toxic compound. The hypercalcaemia is due to increased absorption of calcium from the gastrointestinal tract. In patients on treatment with vitamin D or its metabolites changes in 24-hour urine calcium excretion may be of predictive value.

Sarcoid

Hypercalcaemia is a rare complication in patients with sarcoid. The mechanism for hypercalcaemia in sarcoidosis was in the past attributed to hypersensitivity to all of the actions of cholecalciferol. There is now evidence that it is due to excessive production of 1,25-DHCC. These patients have very low or undetectable serum values of i-PTH and increased values of 1,25-DHCC.

Thyrotoxicosis

Hypercalcaemia may occur in association with hyperthyroidism either as a direct complication or as a manifestation of associated primary hyperparathyroidism. The mechanism of the hypercalcaemia that occurs as a direct complication of hyperthyroidism is not clear.

Milk-alkali syndrome (Milk-drinker's syndrome)

The features of this syndrome are hypercalcaemia with a metabolic alkalosis. The syndrome occurs in patients with peptic ulcer pain who classically have an excessive intake of milk together with an absorbable alkali, and usually also have evidence of previous renal disease. The self-administration, by peptic ulcer patients, of proprietary preparations containing calcium carbonate is a recognized cause of hypercalcaemia and renal failure. The mechanism of the hypercalcaemia would appear to be the combination of an increase in calcium absorption from the intestine together with a diminution in urine calcium excretion, as a result of decreased glomerular ultrafiltration due to the renal disease. The ingestion of an absorbable alkali, such as calcium carbonate, can itself cause renal damage.

Paget's disease of bone

In patients with Paget's disease of bone (osteitis deformans) hypercalcaemia is a very rare complication and virtually only occurs when the patients are immobilized and confined to bed.

Idiopathic hypercalcaemia of infancy

Hypercalcaemia in infancy occurs in a mild and a severe form and these represent two different disease processes:

1. The *mild form* has been attributed to either an excessive dietary intake of vitamin D or an increased sensitivity to this vitamin; it is, however, possible that variations in endogenous faecal calcium excretion may play a role.
2. The *severe form* is rare and constitutes a syndrome characterized by 'elfin-like' facies, mental retardation, osteosclerosis, hypercalcaemia, hypercalciuria, nephrocalcinosis and uraemia. The mechanism of the hypercalcaemia in the severe form is unknown.

Adrenocortical insufficiency

Hypercalcaemia may occur in patients with adrenocortical insufficiency with an incidence comparable to that of hyponatraemia, although it may be the only electrolyte abnormality. The mechanism for the hypercalcaemia is not clearly defined.

Hypocalcaemia

The most common presentation is with paraesthesiae in the hands (finger tips), in the feet and around the mouth. The most striking clinical feature of hypocalcaemia is tetany with carpo-pedal spasms in adults or laryngeal spasm in infants; some patients especially infants present with convulsions. Psychiatric symptoms may occur, the most common of which are anxiety and depression. Chronic hypocalcaemia may be associated with progressive intellectual loss and cataract.

The differential diagnosis of hypocalcaemia is based on the causative mechanism and this can very often be clarified by a careful history and physical examination. Among the points that need to be elucidated are the following:

1. Previous neck surgery.
2. History of gastrointestinal malabsorption.
3. Drug therapy.
4. Vegetarian or vegan diet.
5. Sunshine exposure.

In only a few patients do laboratory investigations play a major differential diagnostic role; they do, however, play a major confirmatory role.

Chronic renal failure

Hypocalcaemia is one of the classic features of chronic renal failure. The continual loss of nephrons in chronic renal failure is associated with a reduction in the formation of 1,25-DHCC. Nephron loss also leads to an inability to excrete phosphorus with a consequent rise in serum concentration. The increase in serum phosphate concentration causes a reduction in ionized calcium concentration which leads to secondary hyperparathyroidism. There has been considerable controversy as to which mechanism is responsible for the osteomalacia and osteitis fibrosa of chronic renal failure. It has recently been shown that serum levels of 1,25-DHCC remain normal until the glomerular filtration rate has fallen to 40 ml/min or less although i-PTH values begin to increase at an early stage of chronic renal failure. This does not, however, mean that it is the inability of the kidney to excrete phosphate that is all important in renal osteodystrophy, as a raised 1,25-DHCC would be the appropriate response to the falling serum calcium associated with phosphate retention. The change in the ratio of PTH to 1,25-DHCC might even shift the response to the falling serum calcium from intestine to bone.

Gastrointestinal disorders

Hypocalcaemia can occur with malabsorption from any cause including coeliac disease, pancreatic disorders, biliary obstruction and following partial gastrectomy. There is no consistent relationship between the severity of the steatorrhea, the degree of hypocalcaemia and/or the occurrence of osteomalacia. Many factors contribute to the defects of calcium metabolism in patients with malabsorption, including intestinal absorption of exogenous vitamin D and the enterohepatic circulation not only of vitamin D metabolites but also calcium. The latter mechanism may be of particular importance in patients with chronic liver disorders. In chronic liver disease the hypocalcaemia is potentially due to a number of mechanisms including low sunlight exposure, low dietary vitamin D intake, interference by bilirubin with skin cholecalciferol synthesis, malabsorption of exogenous and endogenous vitamin D and interruption of the enterohepatic circulation, and diminished hepatic 25-hydroxylase activity.

Hypoparathyroidism

The most common cause of hypoparathyroidism is surgical damage to the parathyroid glands or their blood supply during neck surgery. In these patients the hypocalcaemia is associated with undetectable values of i-PTH.

In some rare patients with hypocalcaemia there may appear to be adequate circulating concentrations of i-PTH. In these patients the hypocalcaemia may represent target tissue unresponsiveness due to a deficiency in the PTH-sensitive adenyl cyclase–cAMP system; a disorder described as *pseudohypoparathyroidism*. The differentiation between the various types of hypoparathyroidism can be made on the basis of changes in urinary cAMP excretion following the administration of exogenous parathyroid extract.

'Nutritional' vitamin-D deficiency

Hypocalcaemia under this heading only occurs in patients who have both a dietary lack of vitamin together with lack of adequate exposure to bright sunshine (ultraviolet light). The major problem is a lack of exposure to ultraviolet light which initiates the primary step in the synthesis of cholecalciferol in the skin.

Neonatal

Neonatal hypocalcaemia can either be of a transient or persistent type. The potential factors involved include:

1. Functional 'immaturity' of parathyroid glands.
2. The calcium to phosphorus ratio of artifical or formula milks. Cow's milk has a high phosphorus content with a low calcium/phosphorus ratio compared with human breast milk; this ratio is of importance in the intestinal absorption mechanism.

Neonatal hypocalcaemia, with tetany or convulsions, may be the first manifestation of primary hyperparathyroidism in the mother. The importance of the diagnosis of the latter disease is that the occurrence of convulsions in a newborn infant justifies the estimation of the mother's serum calcium concentration.

Anticonvulsant drugs

Hypocalcaemia may occur in patients on treatment with diphenylhydantoin or phenobarbital. The mechanism of the latter is hepatic enzyme induction with a consequent disturbance in cholecalciferol metabolism.

Acute pancreatitis

Hypocalcaemia occurs relatively frequently in patients with acute pancreatitis. A variety of mechanisms have been proposed to account for the hypocalcaemia in this disease and include the precipitation of calcium–magnesium salts with fatty acids in areas of fat necrosis, hypoalbuminaemia and a glucagon-induced increase in calcitonin secretion.

Hypomagnesaemia

The mechanism for the hypocalcaemia that frequently accompanies hypomagnesaemia is controversial. Among the postulated mechanisms are a tissue resistance to the action of PTH and a defect in the release or a cleavage block in the secretion of PTH from the parathyroid glands.

Appendix

Normal endocrine reference values and factors for the conversion of conventional to SI units

Throughout the text of this book SI units have been used. This Appendix provides a set of normal reference endocrine values and factors for conversion of conventional units to SI. It is, however, important to stress that in all situations the reader should rely on the reference values supplied by the laboratory that is providing the test services.

Aldosterone (Mol wt 360.45)

SI unit–pmol/ℓ
Conversion factor ng/100 ml $\times$ 27.8 = pmol
Serum:

Less than 1 year	220–2000 pmol/ℓ
1–4 years	70–750 pmol/ℓ
5–9 years	30–400 pmol/ℓ
10–15 years	55–550 pmol/ℓ
Adults	38 to 410 pmol/ℓ

Calcitonin

SI unit–ng/ℓ
Serum:
<80 ng/ℓ

Cortisol (Mol wt 362.47)

SI unit–nmol/ℓ
Conversion factor μg/100 ml $\times$ 27.6 = nmol/ℓ
Serum:
    0900 hours   220–770 nmol/ℓ
    2400 hours   55–250 nmol/ℓ
Urine free:
    Adult females   216–860 nmol/24h
    Adult males   300–1100 nmol/24h
    8-hour overnight excretion   25–220 nmol

1,25-Dihydroxycholecalciferol

See Vitamin D Metabolites

Follicle-stimulating hormone (FSH)

SI unit–U/ℓ
Serum:
    Adult females
        Follicular phase   3–16 U/ℓ
        Mid-cycle phase   12–27 U/ℓ
        Luteal phase   2–16 U/ℓ
        Post-menopausal   40–185 U/ℓ
    Adult males   3–16 U/ℓ
    Children (1 year to puberty)   2.5 U/ℓ

Gonadotrophins

See LH and FSH

Growth hormone

SI unit–mU/ℓ
Serum:
    Adults   less than 10 mU/ℓ

Hydroxyproline (Mol wt 131.13)

SI unit–μmol/24h
Conversion factor mg/24 hours × 7.63 = μmol/24 h
Urine:
    Adults   114–470 μmol/24 h

25-Hydroxyvitamin D

See Vitamin D metabolites

Luteinizing hormone (LH)

SI unit–U/ℓ
Serum:
    Adult females
        Follicular phase   3–45 U/ℓ
        Mid-cycle phase   45–300 U/ℓ
        Luteal phase   3–45 U/ℓ
        Post-menopausal   49–128 U/ℓ
    Adult males   5 to 23 U/ℓ

3-Methoxy-4-hydroxymandelic acid (HMMA)–Also known as VMA (mol wt 197.18)

SI unit–μmol/ℓ or 24 hours
Conversion factor mg/24 h × 5.05 = μmol/24 h
Urine:
    Adults   10–35 μmol/24 h
    Total catecholamines less than 600 nmol/24 h

Oestradiol-17β (Mol wt 272.39)

SI unit–pmol/ℓ
Conversion factor ng/100 ml × 36.5 = pmol/ℓ
Serum:
    Adult females
        Follicular phase   110–370 pmol/ℓ
        Peri-ovulatory phase 370–1470 pmol/ℓ

Luteal phase	180–550 pmol/ℓ
Post-menopausal phase	20–70 pmol/ℓ
Adult males	40–220 pmol/ℓ

Oestriol (total oestrogens) (Mol wt 288.39)

SI unit–nmol/24 h (pregnancy)
       nmol/24 h (non-pregnant)
Conversion factor mg/24 h × 3.47 = nmol/24 h
       μg/24 h × 3.47 = nmol/24 h
Urine:

    Adult females non-pregnant

Follicular phase	25–105 nmol/24 h
Ovulatory mid-cycle peak	140–350 nmol/24 h
Luteal phase	105–350 nmol/24 h
Adult males	25–90 nmol/24 h

17-Oxogenic steroids

SI unit–μmol/24 h
Conversion factor mg/24 h × 3.47 = μmol/24 h

Adult females	14–50 μmol/24 h
Adult males	17–70 μmol/24 h

17-Oxosteroids (Mol wt 288.4 as Dehydroepiandrosterone)

SI unit–μmol/24 h
Conversion factor mg/24 h × 3.47 = μmol/24 h

Adult females	14–60 μmol/24 h
Adult males	20–90 μmol/24 h

Parathyroid hormone

Arbitrary units
Serum:

i-PTH-Carboxyterminal	0.3–1.3 ng/ml*
i-PTH-Aminoterminal	18–40 pg/ml*

*with simultaneous serum calcium concentrations of 2.10 –2.60 mmol/ℓ

Pregnanediol (Mol wt 320.50)

SI unit–μmol/24 h
Conversion factor mg/24 hours × 3.12 = μmol/24 h
Urine:
>   Adult females
>>   Follicular phase   0–1.6 μmol/24 h
>>   Luteal phase   >6 μmol/24 h
>>   Post-menopausal   0.4–2.8 μmol/24 h
>   Adult males   0–3.0 μmol/24 h

Progesterone (Mol wt 318.45)

Si unit–nmol/ℓ
Conversion factor ng/100 ml × 0.03 = nmol/ℓ
Serum:
>   Adult females
>>   Follicular phase   0.6–2.9 nmol/ℓ
>>   Luteal phase   9.5–95 nmol/ℓ
>>   Post-menopausal   0.1–1.0 nmol/ℓ
>   Adult males   0.3–1.3 nmol/ℓ

Prolactin

SI unit–U/ℓ
>   Adult females   25–396 U/ℓ
>   Adult males   5–178 U/ℓ

Testosterone (Mol wt 288.43)

SI unit–nmol/ℓ
Conversion factor μg/100 ml × 34.5 = nmol/ℓ
Serum:
>   Adult females   0.7–2.8 nmol/ℓ
>   Adult males   10.4–34.6 nmol/ℓ

Tri-iodothyronine (Mol wt 651.01)

SI unit–nmol/ℓ
Conversion factor ng/100 ml × 0.015 = nmol/ℓ
Serum:
    Adults   0.8–2.5 nmol/ℓ

Thyroid-stimulating hormone (TSH)

SI unit–mU/ℓ
Serum:
    Adults   1–6 mU/ℓ

Thyroxine (Mol wt 776.93)

SI unit–nmol/ℓ
Conversion facor μg/100 ml × 12.8 = nmol/ℓ
Serum:
    Adults (total)   54–142 nmol/ℓ
    Adults (free)   8.8–23 pmol/ℓ

Vanilmandelic acid (VMA)

See 3-Methoxy-4-hydroxymandelic acid

Vitamin D metabolites
1,25-Dihydroxycholecalciferol

SI unit–pmol/ℓ
Serum:
    Adults   130–240 pmol/ℓ

25-Hydroxyvitamin D
SI unit–nmol/ℓ
Serum:
    Adults   25–95 nmol/ℓ